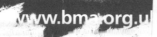
The Primary FRCA:
A Complete Guide to Preparation
and Passing

Acquisitions editor: Melanie Tait
Development editor: Zoë Youd
Production controller: Pauline Sones
Desk editor: Jane Campbell
Cover designer: Greg Harris

The Primary FRCA:
A Complete Guide to
Preparation and Passing

RM Sharpe FRCA
MD Brunner FRCA
SM Yentis MD FRCA*
M Hasan FRCA
PN Robinson FRCA

*Consultant Anaesthetists and Honorary Senior Lecturers,
Imperial College School of Medicine, London*
*Northwick Park and St Mark's Hospitals, Harrow, Middlesex
UK*

*Chelsea and Westminster Hospital, London UK

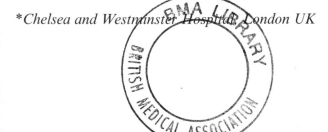

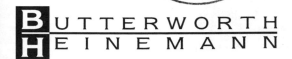

BUTTERWORTH
HEINEMANN

OXFORD AUCKLAND BOSTON JOHANNESBURG MELBOURNE NEW DELHI

Butterworth-Heinemann
Linacre House, Jordan Hill, Oxford OX2 8DP
225 Wildwood Avenue, Woburn, MA 01801–2041

A division of Reed Educational and Professional Publishing Ltd

A member of the Reed Elsevier plc group

First published 2002

British Library Cataloguing in Publication Data
A catalogue record for this book in available from the British Library

Library of Congress Cataloguing in Publication Data
A catalogue record for this book is available from the Library of Congress

ISBN 0 7506 5220 9

For information on all Butterworth-Heinemann publications visit our website at www.bh.com

Printed and bound in Great Britain by MPG Books Ltd, Bodmin, Cornwall

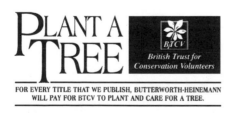

FOR EVERY TITLE THAT WE PUBLISH, BUTTERWORTH-HEINEMANN
WILL PAY FOR BTCV TO PLANT AND CARE FOR A TREE.

Contents

Preface

Reality for the trainee anaesthetist is the sitting and the passing of the FRCA examination within a certain time period. This two-part hurdle has become pivotal to 'seamless' anaesthetic training. The Primary FRCA examination has the distinct ability to swoop down on unsuspecting victims early on in their career, finding them totally unprepared and often panic-stricken. This can be compared to the definition of the sound of distant elephants: *you only realize the rumbling has become much louder when you are about to be trampled on.* This book attempts to avoid that scenario for the candidate.

Therefore, we are concerned with covering all aspects of the Primary examination in this text including preparation and examination technique. Guidance notes at the beginning of each chapter offer advice on the nature of each component of the examination.

However, there is no substitute for diligent preparation. We hope that the advice and questions offered in this book will help the trainee study confidently, prepare from the enclosed practice questions and pass the examination.

We trust that the readers will forgive us the odd moment of humour and the occasional idiosyncratic MCQ question.

Roger Sharpe
Michael Brunner
Maan Hasan
Steve Yentis
Neville Robinson

1 Candidates, examiners and the examination

The Primary FRCA (Fellowship of the Royal College of Anaesthetists) examination should be taken by well-prepared candidates with a positive attitude who understand the whole examination. This introductory chapter will discuss the necessary background preparation and revision strategies necessary for the candidate. This knowledge will advantage the candidate and put them 'ahead of the field' in comparison to less well prepared candidates.

There are many ways in which prospective candidates can improve their chances of passing the exam: general support; improving their examination technique; and acquiring and improving practical skills and knowledge. General support is often overlooked but is extremely important. It includes preparing everybody around you that you are going to be under great strain in the near future. It also includes teaming up with fellow trainees and pooling resources wherever possible. You will need to rely on each other for examination practice. You also need to talk about the exam to your more senior colleagues so that the whole department is right behind you. Working for exams in isolation is very difficult. Improving your exam technique involves planning your revision and knowing and practising the various parts of the exams. Knowing what to expect and when to expect it can make a huge difference to your performance on the day. Lastly, the acquisition of skills and knowledge means the subject itself must be covered and fitted into the examination framework – you need to get used to thinking in an 'exam-orientated' way from quite early on, so that each encounter with patients or colleagues can be exploited to gain the learning potential from it.

THE FRCA EXAMINATION

The FRCA examination is in two parts. About 700 candidates sit each part of the exam per year. Detailed regulations for the FRCA are published by the Royal College and are easily accessible via the college website at http://www.rcoa.ac.uk. Prospective candidates are advised to obtain these and study them well. In brief, candidates may sit the Primary if they have full or provisional General Medical Council registration, have registered with The College as a postgraduate anaesthetic trainee and have completed at least 1 year's satisfactory anaesthetic training as an SHO in an approved hospital (College Tutors often advise that 18 months experience is preferable prior to sitting the examination). The dates of the exam sittings are usually published a year in advance. Candidates are advised to make sure they meet the practical requirements and deadline for applications.

Many candidates who fail the examination have taken it when they are not really ready. Only four attempts at the Primary are allowed, so it is important that you only sit the exam if you are fully prepared.

The structure of the examination

The exam consists of three sections: a multiple choice questions (MCQ) paper, the vivas and the Objectively Structured Clinical Examinations (OSCEs) (the last two together constitute the 'oral' part of the exam). Only those candidates who pass the MCQ paper can go on to sit the orals.

The Primary examination tests:

- The fundamentals of clinical anaesthetic practice including equipment and resuscitation
- The fundamental principles of anatomy, physiology, pharmacology, physics, clinical measurement and statistics as is appropriate for the discipline of anaesthesia
- The skills and attitudes appropriate to the above level of training

As can be seen, this definition serves to set the scene for what is required of the candidate. The exam essentially functions as a screening tool to help identify anaesthetic trainees who are suitable to progress to a specialist registrar rotation.

The examiners

Be reassured the examiners are normal people who become examiners because they feel it is important to maintain standards of practice of anaesthesia. Being an examiner is generally hard work and requires great commitment. Although many examiners are academic anaesthetists, there is not a minimum quota and you could find yourself face to face with a professor from a teaching centre or a consultant from a district general hospital. These days examiners are offered a great deal of guidance and support and there is ongoing assessment and audit of *their* performance, so increasingly examiners are coming under similar stresses and pressures to the candidates. There is no doubt that some examiners are more 'hawkish' whilst others are more 'dovish', but (i) that's true of life anyway, and (ii) pairing of hawks with doves and the move towards standardizing the exam should minimize any effect this has on an individual candidate's results.

Examiners are very aware of candidate anxiety and have great empathy with the candidates. They also feel the anxiety of the 'prolonged silence' and, contrary to public belief, want the candidates to do well. However, a candidate who will not speak cannot pass – in vivas and the OSCEs the candidates must talk fluently and not just in single words. Examiners shouldn't have to drag information out of the candidate.

The Royal College allows observers to attend the orals to demonstrate the open nature of the exam and to aid the training of future candidates. They are allowed to 'sit in' during the vivas and OSCE stations. They are not allowed to get involved in any candidate's actual performance and the candidate is advised not to be distracted by observers and to speak only to the examiners.

Marking

The same basic method of marking is used for all parts of the examination and is based on a fairly narrow range of possible marks:

0   Veto; the candidate is absent (or their answer is) and therefore cannot score at all
1   The candidate has failed poorly
1+ The candidate has failed, although only just; it is still possible to pass the examination provided the candidate scores 2 or 2+ in all the other sections of the exam
2   The candidate has passed
2+ This score is only given if the candidate is being considered for a prize, for which a 2+ in every part of the examination at the first sitting is required.

All parts of the examination and their answers are subject to careful scrutiny in order to reject questions that are too easy or too difficult (e.g. every candidate passes or fails them respectively), whilst retaining for further use those questions which can identify the good candidates from those who fail the whole exam (i.e. good discriminatory questions).

PREPARING FOR THE EXAM

There is no alternative to revision. To prepare for the exam, you need to acquire or consolidate a number of things:

* *Knowledge* – pretty obvious on the face of it, but surprisingly often overlooked.
* *Practical skills* – you may be tested on these in action or simply by your ability to describe how you do certain procedures.
* *Problem-solving* – the ability to interpret information and suggest courses of action is one thing we tend to be groomed towards during our long under- and postgraduate training, and we rely on this every time we face a patient.
* *Examination technique* – the ability to persuade the

examiners how fantastic you really are underneath that quivering, blubbering mess that faces them.

- *Attitudes* – harder to define; basically you have to be able to demonstrate that you are a caring, professional and decisive sort of person who can make the appropriate decisions in the context of the whole patient. The best source of inspiration for this is usually your own department and its members (who should influence you positively but may influence negatively in this regard).

Planning your revision

Most experienced examination teachers advise some sort of plan for revision. This ensures you cover all the required ground and allows you to pace yourself and highlight your progress which inspires a sense of achievement and confidence. The first task in drawing up a revision plan is to decide when to start. The choice must vary depending on the individual as you don't want to peak too early but on the other hand it would be nice to peak at some point! We'd suggest a total of 6–8 months starting with general background reading and ending with a period of about 10 weeks, of 'intensive' revision.

What to cover

The syllabus is published by the College and available on the College website, and you must get a copy and study it well. The subjects are listed by major subject headings and the topics within them. These may be used to draw up a revision plan and detailed guidance is included on most topics. The Syllabus headings are:

- Anaesthesia and resuscitation
- Anatomy
- Physiology and biochemistry
- Pharmacology
- Physics and clinical measurement
- Basic statistics
- Skills

Getting going

One of the hardest parts of revising is getting started. Essentially once you have a revision plan and knowing the speed at which you personally work you need to set a date on which 'my revision begins' and stick to it. Avoid delaying tactics such as 'I will wait just another week'. Avoid fooling yourself that you are 'revising' without actually doing anything of the sort, e.g. by compiling complicated three-dimensional revision timetables with six colours taking several hours of hard 'work'. Avoid spending fortunes buying every available textbook which you will never have time to read let alone digest the facts.

As with the above examples, there is no real alternative to hard work. There are, however, a number of useful ways in which you can get into the frame of things:

1. Draw up a sensible revision plan which you know you can work to and use this as a guide for the entire period leading up to the exam.
2. Start compiling a list of those vital facts beloved of anaesthetic examinations: drug details and doses; physiochemical drug data; physics and physiology formulae; composition of intravenous fluids; physiological data; etc. You'll find that the list grows as you look around for more things to include. This list can become a major tool in your revision programme and putting it together is a good way of getting yourself to think about the various topics relatively easily.
3. Book yourself onto a preparatory course. There are several of these and they are often timed around the exams. However, courses are notorious for giving a false sense of revision security ('How's the revising going?' 'Fine thanks, I'm going on a course'.).

With all these methods of getting going and also with the main revision itself, it is important not to be too ambitious with your aims, since allowing yourself to slip can be very demoralizing as the amount of work required to 'catch up' increases in front of your eyes. Having made your plans and set your targets, though, it is vital that you be absolutely rigid with sticking to them.

Pacing yourself

Once you have a list of topics to revise, you have to pace your progress to ensure you cover the whole ground. If you give yourself enough time, it should be possible not only to go through the complete plan, but to do so several times thus consolidating previous revision. To set your pace you can either start out with an open mind and see how far you get in the first week or two, or alternatively see how long it takes you to get through say, 10–20 individual topics. You can then concentrate on slowing down or speeding up as appropriate. Aim at going through the entire list at least twice and more often if possible. Of course, nearer the time it would probably be worth leaving out the more obscure topics and concentrating on the more important ones.

You must give yourself an allotted time every day for proper revision. This is best measured in hours and 1–2 hour blocks are probably the minimum units; most people find less than an hour is simply too short a period to allow any constructive revision. Thus for example your average evening could be divided into two 1.5 hour sessions with a break in between. Do not stay up into the early hours of the morning revising. It's important to set yourself the task in advance (e.g. deciding on the way home how many hours you'll do that evening) because you can then plan your evening around the revision sessions. As already mentioned, you should be realistic in setting your targets and not be too ambitious (after all, you are an anaesthetist, not a surgeon!), and you should be absolutely determined to achieve however many sessions you have set yourself. The 'I'll just start and see how it goes' approach generally doesn't work as well and is not as good for charting your progress. Setting yourself a target and achieving it does great things for your confidence too, but try to resist the temptation of celebrating by having the next week off. Having said that, you may need to bribe yourself with various rewards for

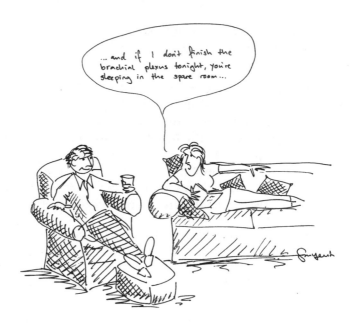

accomplishing the set task(s) of the day, especially at the beginning.

REVISION

Once you've cleared the social decks, arranged psychological support, enlisted friends, family and colleagues, promised yourself specific treats (or beatings) to spur you on and drawn up a plan for the next several months, it's time to sit down and go through the material. This time must be free of distractions. Breaks are also important and try to make a conscious effort to relax and clear your mind during them. Once it comes down to the subjects themselves, there are many ways of going through them. To break up the revision process, try to change from one method to another every now and then.

Structured revision

1. Reading books

Books are invaluable sources of information, largely because someone else has taken the trouble to sift out the rubbish and present the useful material in a user-friendly way. However, reading can (i) take up a lot of time and (ii) be done whilst you are half-asleep with very little benefit to you (how often have you read a whole page only to realize you haven't taken in a single word?). Finally, beware the dangers of having too many books, as you will not be able to read them all and the more authorities you consult, the more different opinions you obtain. Nonetheless, books are a very useful adjunct to revision. There is an increasing number of anaesthetic textbooks from which to choose; the best guides are the opinions of fellow trainees. Try and buy books that you will be able to read and use expensive 'reference' books from the library.

2. Making notes from various sources

Whilst having a large and comprehensive series of authoritative notes on the whole syllabus is certainly attractive, by the time you've finished the task, you've (i) got another wad of paperwork to read and (ii) used up a large proportion of your time. Borrowing others' notes is generally a waste of time.

3. Writing cue cards

Although similar to note-making, this seems more efficient in terms of use of time, since all you need to write on each card are the bare essentials for each topic (in fact, this is the way some people take notes anyway). Each term written then acts as a prompt rather than a source of information in its own right. This style of annotating goes well with viva and OSCE practice.

4. Writing answer plans

Answer plans are one of the best ways of preparing answers for the orals, since it allows you to practice angling a response towards a directed question. Many questions fall into groups of similar types and can be tackled in similar ways as in the examples below.

(a) How would you manage a patient with a specified condition requiring surgery?
Answer plan:
Introduction: incidence/background of condition
Effects of the condition on pre-existing state
Effects of anaesthesia/surgery on condition
Preoperative: general and specific assessment
treatment, stabilization and premedication
Peroperative: check equipment/monitoring/staff
induction/maintenance/recovery fluids/
position/other
Postoperative: analgesia/special care/fluids

(b) Tell me about drug ...
Answer plan:
Class of drug/mode of action
Uses/indications
Presentation/storage/presentation/physical properties
Administration/dose
Pharmacodynamics (effects of the drug on the body –
go through the systems)
CVS, RS, CNS, GI tract, endocrine,
musculoskeletal, placenta, skin, eye
Pharmacokinetics (effects of the body on the drug)
absorption, distribution, metabolism, excretion
Side effects/adverse reactions

(c) How would you perform a specific nerve block?
Answer plan:
Indications/contraindications/consent
Technique: awake vs. asleep, asepsis, position,
landmarks, approach, end-point, needle, nerve
stimulator

Local anaesthetic: agent, concentration, volume
Effects of procedure (i.e. desirable ones)
Complications (i.e. undesirable ones)

It is useful to draw up answer plans once you have gone through a topic in its entirety (e.g. dural taps), you can then set yourself a specific examination approach to the topic, e.g. 'What factors increase the likelihood of accidental dural tap' or 'How would you manage an accidental dural tap'. Another useful thing to do with answer plans is to show them to each other and to senior colleagues in your department. For example, if three of you quickly write out a couple of plans on the same subject, you can compare them and see which bits each of you have missed out. Showing them to more senior anaesthetists may produce useful tips and identify omissions as well.

Many anaesthetic answer plans can incorporate the surgical sieve. For example, use the following sieve to list the causes of difficult intubation.

Congenital
Acquired:
Trauma
Infective
Neurological
Vascular
Inflammatory
Neoplastic
Endocrine
Metabolic
Iatrogenic
Deficiency
Idiopathic
Psychological

5. *Diagrams*

Make a list of those diagrams you must know but always forget, e.g. oxyhaemoglobin dissociation curve, brachial plexus, cross-section of the neck, etc. One by one, draw out the

the diagram from memory (such as it is), then look at the real version in a book or your notes, then draw it out again.

6. Reading journals

It is worth flicking through the last few issues of the main anaesthetic journals, looking for good reviews and editorials. These will give you comprehensive and up to date viewpoints of the topics covered.

7. Give a talk

As part of your departmental meetings/teaching you may be required to give a presentation. Use this as a revision opportunity as the presentation will encourage you to read the subject 'in-depth' and to produce a plan which is similar to the answer plan method. Giving a presentation about a subject helps you to verbalize your knowledge which is especially important for the oral parts of the examination.

8. Courses

You should always try to get on to a course if you can. It will stimulate or scare you into revision. Part of their benefit is derived from mingling with others in a similar position, and swapping tips. However, courses are notorious for giving a false sense of revision security and shouldn't substitute other types of revision.

Courses are generally either 'day-release' or 2–3 weeks of continuous lectures/study. You will need to decide which is suited to you. For example, a day-release course over several months leading up to the examination stopping a month or so before the examination will give you a welcome regular break from hospital work and give you more time to get yourself into the examination mood, whereas a 1–3 week intensive 'crammer' course suits some better by demanding and delivering more within a short period of time. You may need to plan well in advance since you may have to negotiate study leave with other hopefuls in your department.

Unstructured revision

This term includes other opportunities occurring throughout the day which can be used to increase and consolidate your knowledge.

1. Operating theatre lists

Take time to examine every bit of equipment in your anaesthetic room, theatre, cupboard, etc. Keep a notebook to list the things that you don't understand so you can look these subjects up later. Similarly, every time you do a case, imagine you're answering a question on what complications may occur, which anaesthetic techniques are especially suitable. If there's someone with you, get them involved.

2. Odd minutes

Remember that list of useful numbers, equations, etc., that you drew up when you started getting into an examination frame of mind? Keep the list with you and during odd moments of spare time go through it testing yourself on each item, writing out the correct answer each time you get it wrong. This will help you to have these facts at your fingertips during the examination which is impressive from the examiners' point of view and allows you to handle related MCQs with greater confidence.

3. Practice answers

Whenever you have a spare moment, practise answering questions; you can make them up in your head or carry a list of 'topics du jour' around with you. This can easily be done on the way home, over meals or even in the bath.

4. Be inquisitive

Preparing for an examination is also an excuse to go through your department's protocols, guidelines, storage rooms, etc., and ask your senior colleagues (and drug reps!) about recent developments, reports and what's topical.

5. Practical skills

Try hard to develop good practical skills – pay particular attention when watching others doing procedures and try to criticize them (to yourself). Be conscious of trying to achieve perfection when doing them yourself. For example, when you perform a regional block or invasive technique, describe to yourself the anatomy, technique, etc., as you do it. Developing good attitudes is harder but look around and watch/talk to your colleagues; identify the attributes that impress you and adopt them, whilst rejecting those that don't.

6. Good habits

Get used to referring to drugs by their generic names, not their trade names. Saying 'Diprivan' or 'Zofran' in an oral examination is like a red rag to a bull to most examiners. Write out the proper name every time you prescribe the drug or record its use on the anaesthetic chart. Also, swallow your nationalistic pride and use the recommended international names for drugs.

7. Journals

Always carry a good review article or two around with you. When you have a break and you can't face the above methods, go through one. By using your time employing different approaches, you're more likely to break the monotony and thus avoid boredom.

SUMMARY

You will of course pick and choose what you want to do (if anything) from the above suggestions, but whatever you do decide upon, there are some general points which really must apply if you are to give yourself the best chance at going into the examinations well prepared. Ensuring that you have general support at home and at work; planning your revision and dividing the tasks into attainable chunks; sticking to your plan like glue; building in breaks and treats; and above all changing the methods you use day-by-day or even session-by-session to maintain variety, will at the very least give a feeling of structure to your life at a time when the stresses and pressures are building up to their worst. If you have found other techniques or strategies to be particularly useful for you, then you must stick with them.

Each subsequent chapter has advice on how to prepare and pass the individual aspects of the examination. There are two complete examinations in each section for you to work through.

2 The Multiple Choice Questions (MCQs)

Pass these and you are on the way to the next phase of the examination. Don't fail badly (score 1 or 0) or you will be deferred until the next examination! MCQs test breadth and depth of knowledge so attempt to learn the whole syllabus.

This component of the examination consists of a 3 hour examination of 90 questions. Each question has a 'stem' and five 'branches' which are either true or false. The MCQs test knowledge of the basic sciences, and there are 30 pharmacology, 30 physiology and biochemistry, and 30 physics and clinical measurement questions.

MARKING

Before talking about the overall strategy of answering the MCQ paper, it's worth going over the marking system so you can put things into context. A negative marking system operates, whereby a correct answer to each branch of a question earns a mark but an incorrect one loses a mark; thus each question carries a possible range of marks from –5 to +5. No answer, of course, attracts no points. The MCQ paper therefore has the unique and rather dubious claim to fame of being the only part of the examination in which it is possible to achieve a mark of –100%! Candidates are required to obtain a minimum mark in the MCQ paper in order to sit the orals, which is calculated as follows.

All the candidates' actual scores (percentages) are added up and the mean is calculated (the scores are virtually always normally distributed). The mean score is then tweaked according to the scores obtained from specific 'discriminator' questions, which indicate how the cohort of candidates as a whole have performed. These discriminators are scattered throughout the paper and have been found to predict overall performance closely. Analysis of the discriminators enables the mean score to be adjusted upward or downward by a small amount (usually less than 1%) to compensate for the general level of the cohort. Thus, for example, an average candidate will not lose out just because there happens to be an exceptionally clever number of candidates that year and the mean score is a bit higher than usual. The 'adjusted' score then becomes the pass mark for that particular examination. Although the adjustment may be a fraction of a percent, the correction may affect a significant number of candidates since so many are clustered around the mean value. So, all those rumours about what the pass mark actually is for the MCQ don't really cover the whole story: the pass mark varies from sitting to sitting although it usually hovers around or slightly under 50%. Aim for better than 50%!

How do the actual percentages get converted to the 1, 1+, 2 and 2+ scheme? Easy! Candidates scoring the pass mark receive the final MCQ mark of 2, whilst those who achieve more than one standard deviation above this get a 2+. Those within one standard deviation below the pass mark get a 1+ and those below one standard deviation get a 1. Those who run from the examination room after 30 s of the examination in a state of despair and gloom get a 0 and are 'eliminated', in the words of the Royal College of Anaesthetists, along with those scoring a 1.

The rather complicated scheme described above is an amazing example of the efforts being made to mark the MCQs fairly and properly, and is a mixture of complex mathematical calculation and pragmatism. The system works and is constantly under review.

TECHNIQUE

The crucial aspect of answering MCQs is to make sure you **read the question and its stem**, as it's very easy to recognize a few key words in a question and jump to (erroneous) conclusions about the actual nature of the question. We are all generally very good at recognizing patterns without taking in the detail, hence the ease with which 'does' is mistaken for 'does not', 'hypo-' for 'hyper-', and so on. Similarly, it's easy to confuse similarly sounding drugs, such a chlorpromazine and chlorpropramide. These simple mistakes can be disastrous and result in a score of −5 instead of +5 for a particular question. It often helps to read each stem as a continuation of the question. For example, if the question is 'Atropine causes'; followed by (A) bradycardia; (B) sweating; (C) miosis; etc., then read to yourself 'Atropine causes bradycardia' when answering A; 'Atropine causes sweating' when answering B; 'Atropine causes miosis' when answering C; etc. Otherwise, it is easy to lose track of the thread of each question, especially if the question is a long one. Beware words like 'commonly', 'may', etc., it can be hard to quantify just how frequent an event has to be in order to qualify for vague adjectives but it's also hard for the examiners to compile questions and they also have to make difficult decisions. If stuck as to whether the correct answer to a possibly ambiguous question is true or false, before leaving the question alone it may sometimes be worth thinking 'what answer are they actually after'? For example, it is generally advised that propofol should be avoided in epileptic patients because it has been associated with postoperative convulsions and the Committee on the Safety of Medicines has issued a warning on this association. However, not all epileptic patients have problems after propofol and it has even been successfully used to treat status epilepticus. Thus the statement 'Propofol may be safely used in epileptic patients' is strictly speaking correct since it may be used safely. However, the question is more likely to be false than true since the examiners are more likely to be seeking your knowledge that propofol should probably not be used routinely in epileptics, than more detailed knowledge about complicated risk/benefit analysis of treatments in status epilepticus. This kind of ambiguity, which favours the less well-informed candidate over the 'know-all', is rare given the ability of examiners to analyse the pattern of answers, detect bad questions and remove them.

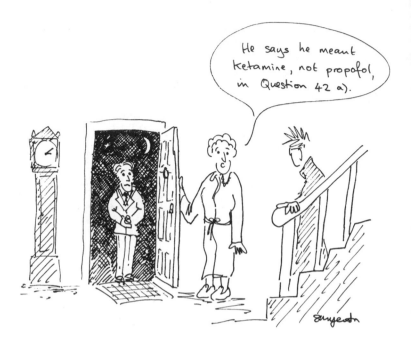

There are countless theories circulating about the best strategic way to tackle MCQs. With luck, you will have evolved a successful strategy for yourself by now (and that is the important bit; what works for someone else may not be right for you) as you will have sat MCQs throughout your undergraduate training, but it should be possible to improve your marks by changing your approach, as described below. Even if you feel relatively comfortable with MCQs, you will have probably never formally tried different methods of actually answering them. Do try out the following exercise – after all you have nothing to lose except a couple of hours – but be disciplined. This means making yourself answer each question as if it were a real exam, including writing down your answers. This is vital since we all tend to get bored during this kind of examination practice and it is tempting to be half-hearted if you know it is only a practice run.

The first step in devising a strategy for answering MCQs is

to consider all parts of whole questions as separate questions, which can then be divided into several categories:

1. *Easy* – you know you know the answer. You can expect to answer almost all of the questions (i.e. > 90%) in this category correctly.
2. *Pretty sure* – you know the subject reasonably well and although not certain, are quite confident of the correct answer, or at least have a pretty good idea. You should still get 70–90% of questions in this category correct, the large range reflecting the broad definition of this category.
3. *Informed guess* – you don't really know, but have enough background knowledge to judge whether a particular answer is more likely to be correct or incorrect. You should still get about 50–70% of these questions correct (i.e. more than half), although there will be lots of incorrect answers as well.
4. *No idea* – answering this category of questions requires a true guess each time; you, therefore, have a 50% chance of guessing it right and will average a score of 0.
5. *Know too much* – these questions are infuriating because although you may know the topic pretty well, you just can't tell which answer is required because of the way in which the question is structured or worded. This type of question should be in a minority since particularly ambiguous or poorly discriminatory questions should be weeded out by the continuous monitoring already mentioned.

The next step is to practise answering MCQ papers in strict order in the manner described above, writing your answers on a separate piece of paper. First, draw five columns down the page and label them 1–5 at the top. Next, go through the paper but for now, only answer those questions in category 1, putting your answers in column 1. Now, go through the paper again answering only those questions in category 2, putting your answers in column 2, and so on, until you have forced yourself to answer all of the questions in the paper, i.e. you've gone through the paper five times. Make sure you read each question properly each time – you will probably be surprised just how many misreading errors you pick up during your repeated runs through. Having worked through the entire paper you should now have a list of your answers identifiable as belonging to the various categories 1–5. Now, mark your answers, applying the traditional marking system. Mark each answer in turn, but when you finish, add up the marks separately for the different categories, giving you five separate scores at the bottom of the five columns. Now, here comes the really clever bit: look at your score for only the category 1 questions, and see how your score changes as you add the scores from successive categories of question. Most people's scores improve as they increase the number of questions answered, at least up until category 3 questions. Forcing yourself to answer category 4 and 5 questions could go either way; you will need to repeat the exercise several times using different practice papers to determine which stopping point is best for you. If you find that forcing yourself to answer category 4 questions consistently improves your score, it is probably because your answers are not true guesses, a concept which most of us to find hard to accept (see below). In fact, this approach may even help you by forcing you to decide whether a particular question belongs to category 1, 2, 3, 4 or 5 and therefore whether you should attempt an answer or not.

The above approach does take a bit of time, but is worth it since scores can increase by up to a third although most increases are more modest and some people's score actually goes down using this approach. It is also possible, of course, that any improvement is simply a reflection of the amount of MCQ practice involved, rather than any specific change in technique. Also, it can be difficult overcoming your natural aversion to 'guessing', although what we tend to remember as a guess may not actually refer to the true situation. The trouble is, any question with an element of guess-work gets stored in our memory in one of two ways, depending on whether the answer turns out to be right or wrong, and this reinforces our built in conviction that guessing is bad. For example, when discovering our answer was wrong we curse and say 'I shouldn't have guessed', but if it was right, we say to ourselves 'That wasn't really a guess; I knew it all the time'. Whichever approach you eventually go for, you should always start with the questions you have the best chance of getting right, i.e. starting with category 1 and then going through the categories in order, so that if you do run out of time, at least you have already scored the bulk of your points.

We should point out here that successive statements from the Royal College of Anaesthetists have stressed the importance of not guessing MCQs. This is based on the examination results that they have obtained. It may be that this conclusion has been reached from analysis of discriminatory questions mentioned at the beginning of this chapter, but we urge you to try the above technique at least a few times before abandoning it. There have even been published studies supporting the more-is-better approach.

One further practical point: always allow yourself enough time (about 10–15 min) to transfer your answers to the computer card, since you won't score anything if you don't do this. Some advocate doing this as you go along (e.g. answering all category 1 questions and transferring them, then going through category 2 and so on); alternatively you could leave transferring your answers until you've finished – although if you are one of those people who always run out of time in MCQ papers, perhaps you should consider transferring them as you go along. Transferring itself requires particular care and attention. Make sure you check the question number on the paper with the corresponding number on the computer card at regular intervals, say every 10 questions or so. Transferring answers is also a good opportunity for one final check of each question and answer (still looking for those misreadings).

CONCLUSION

Once you have found your best technique for answering the questions, there are really only two ways to revise for the MCQ paper: practise MCQs and improve your general depth of knowledge by general revision. We cannot do the revision for you but we can provide you with examination standard practice papers and we enclose two in this section. There are a few 'rogue' questions included in an attempt to make the topic less tedious and to help you to remember that there is more to life than examinations. Good luck!

MCQ Examination Paper A

1. **For laminar flow, the flow rate of a fluid along a tube is directly proportional to**
   A. The viscosity of the fluid
   B. The density of the fluid
   C. The length of the tube
   D. The radius of the tube
   E. The square root of the molecular weight of the fluid

2. **Regarding intravenous infusions**
   A. The initial loading dose is dependent on the volume of distribution of the drug
   B. The maintenance infusion rate equals the desired plasma concentration divided by the clearance
   C. Propofol obeys a multi-compartment pharmacokinetic model
   D. At steady state the volume of distribution of propofol is 12 ml/kg body weight
   E. The context sensitive half-time of a drug is dependent on the length of time of the infusion

3. **The partial pressure of oxygen at sea level is**
   A. 21.3 kPa in dry air
   B. 149 mmHg in humidified inspired air at 37°C
   C. 13.3 kPa in the alveolus
   D. 14.5 p.s.i. in inspired gas in a patient breathing 100% oxygen
   E. 40 mmHg higher in the base of the lung than the apex

1. **FFFFF**
   For laminar flow, flow rate (F) is proportional to the pressure gradient across the tube (P) and the fourth power of the radius (r^4). It is inversely proportional to the length of the tube (l) and the viscosity of the fluid. This relationship is described by Poiseuille's equation:

   $$F = \frac{P\pi\, r^4}{8\eta l}$$

2. **TFTFT**
   Loading dose = $V_d \times C_p$, where V_d is the volume of distribution and C_p is the desired plasma concentration of the drug. Maintenance dose = Cl $\times$ C_p, i.e. ml/min $\times$ mg/ml, where Cl is the clearance. At steady state the volume of distribution of propofol is 12 l/kg body weight.

3. **TTTTF**
   Atmospheric pressure is 101.3 kPa, 760 mmHg or 14.5 p.s.i. The partial pressure of oxygen in the air is 21%. 21% of 101.3 kPa is 21.3 kPa. Inspired air is fully saturated with water vapour. At 37°C, the saturated vapour pressure of water is 47 mmHg (6.25 kPa). Therefore at this temperature the partial pressure of oxygen is 21/100 $\times$ (760 – 47) or 149 mmHg or 21/100 $\times$ (101.3 – 6.25) or 19.96 kPa. The alveolar partial pressure of oxygen is determined by the alveolar gas equation: $P_AO_2 = P_IO_2 - P_ACO_2/R$ (where P_AO_2 is the alveolar partial pressure of oxygen, P_IO_2 is the partial pressure of inspired oxygen, P_ACO_2 is the partial pressure of alveolar carbon dioxide and R is the respiratory quotient). P_IO_2 is 21/100 $\times$ (101.3 – 6.25) or 19.96 kPa. P_ACO_2 is approximately 5.33 kPa and R is 0.8. Therefore, $P_AO_2 = $ 19.96 – 5.33/0.8 = 13.3 kPa. The partial pressure of oxygen is 40 mmHg higher in the apex of the lung than the base.

4. **Regarding antibiotics**
   A. Ciprofloxacin is a beta-lactam antibiotic
   B. Meropenem is inactive against Gram-positive bacteria
   C. Vancomycin is effective against MRSA
   D. Clavulanic acid is an antibiotic which is active against
      Haemophilus influenzae
   E. Ceftazidine is active against *Pseudomonas aeruginosa*

5. **Regarding units of pressure, 1 atmosphere equals**
   A. 760 mmHg
   B. 7600 torr
   C. 1.013 N/m^2
   D. 101.3 kPa
   E. 1033 cmH$_2$O

6. **Regarding drugs which effect clotting**
   A. Warfarin reduces the concentration of clotting factors
      II, VII, IX and X
   B. The effect of warfarin is increased by amiodarone
   C. Aprotinin inhibits plasmin
   D. Heparin is a polypeptide
   E. Streptokinase inhibits plasmin

4. **FFTFT**
Ciprofloxacin is a quinolone. Meropenem is a carbapenem. It is active against both Gram-positive and Gram-negative bacteria. Clavulanic acid is not an antibiotic. It is added to amoxycillin (co-amoxiclav) as it is an inhibitor of beta lactamase. Ceftazidine is a cephalosporin which is active against *Pseudomonas aeruginosa*.

5. **TFFTT**
The torr is numerically the same as the mmHg. Unlike the mmHg, however, the torr is independent of such variables as the density of mercury at different temperatures and pressures. A force of 1 newton (N) acting over an area of 1 square metre (m^2) is 1 pascal (Pa). 1 kPa equals 7.5 mmHg which equals 10.2 cmH_2O. As 760 mmHg equals 1 atm it follows that 1 atm is 101.3 kPa, 1.013×10^5 Pa and 1033 cmH_2O.

6. **TTTFF**
Reduced vitamin K is required in the synthesis by the liver of clotting factors II, VII, IX and X. Warfarin inhibits the reduction of vitamin K, thereby reducing the concentration of these clotting factors. Warfarin is 99% bound to albumin. Amiodarone, as well as non-steroidal anti-inflammatory drugs (NSAIDs) and oral hypoglycaemics displace warfarin from albumin, increasing both the concentration of free drug and its effect. Aprotinin inhibits the breakdown of fibrin clots by plasmin. On the other hand, streptokinase catalyses the formation of plasmin from plasminogen, resulting in the breakdown of fibrin clots. Heparin is a mucopolysaccharide.

7. **Regarding dead space in adult lungs**
    A. Anatomical dead space is determined by measuring the volume of expired carbon dioxide per unit time
    B. Fowler's method measures expired oxygen
    C. The normal anatomical dead space is 150 ml
    D. Nitrous oxide increases the anatomical dead space
    E. Bohr's method measures anatomical dead space

8. **Regarding gas cylinders**
    A. An oxygen cylinder has a black body and black and white quartered shoulders
    B. The pressure in a full entonox cylinder is the same as in a full oxygen cylinder
    C. The Tare weight is the weight of an empty cylinder
    D. In the UK the filling ratio of a nitrous oxide cylinder is 0.67
    E. Carbon dioxide cylinders contain carbon dioxide as a liquid

9. **Regarding pressures (mmHg) within blood vessels**
    A. The pressure in the right ventricle is 25/0
    B. The pressure in the pulmonary artery is 25/8
    C. The pulmonary capillary wedge pressure is approximately 10
    D. The left atrial pressure is greater than the right atrial pressure
    E. The left ventricular diastolic pressure is 10 mmHg greater than the right ventricular diastolic pressure

10. **Regarding intravenous colloids**
    A. The pH of both gelofusin and haemaccel is physiological
    B. 4.5% human albumin solution (HAS) contains more sodium than gelofusine
    C. Gelofusine contains 6.25 mmol/l of calcium
    D. 40% of a dose of hetastarch is excreted unchanged in the urine within 24 h
    E. 1 ml of 20% albumin solution contains 200 mg of albumin

7. **FFTFF**
   Bohr's method measures physiological dead space and involves the measurement of expired carbon dioxide. Bohr's method assumes that all the expired carbon dioxide comes from the alveolus and determines the volume of lung that does not eliminate carbon dioxide. Fowler's method determines anatomical dead space by measuring expired nitrogen following a breath of 100% oxygen. Nitrous oxide has no effect on dead space.

8. **FTTFT**
   An oxygen cylinder has a black body and white shoulders. The pressure in full oxygen and entonox cylinders is 1980 lb/in² or 137 × 100 kPa. The filling ratio is the weight of gas in the cylinder divided by the weight of water the cylinder could hold when full. In the UK the filling ratio is 0.75 whereas in the tropics it is 0.67.

9. **TTTTF**
   The pressure in the left atrium is about 5 mmHg while it is about 2 mmHg in the right atrium. The diastolic pressure in both the left and right ventricles is approximately zero.

10. **TFFTT**
    You have to learn the contents of all the fluids that you give. Several textbooks have tables making comparison between the fluids easier. The pH of gelofusin and haemaccel is 7.4 and 7.3, respectively. Haemaccel contains 6.25 mmol/l of calcium, while gelofusin contains very little.

11. Cortisol
    A. Decreases fatty acid synthesis
    B. Reduces gluconeogenesis
    C. Increases lipolysis
    D. Reduces DNA synthesis
    E. Increases protein catabolism

12. Concerning breathing systems
    A. The Lack breathing attachment is a Mapleson A
    B. The Bain breathing attachment is a Mapleson D
    C. In a Mapleson A system the fresh gas is delivered at the patient end
    D. The adjustable pressure limiting (APL) valve is situated at the patient end in a Magill breathing circuit
    E. The APL valve is situated at the anaesthetic machine end in the Lack breathing system

13. Central venous pressure (CVP)
    A. The x descent follows the c wave
    B. The y descent occurs after opening of the tricuspid valve
    C. The c wave and x descent occur during ventricular systole
    D. The y descent precedes the a wave
    E. The c wave corresponds to closure of the tricuspid valve

14. Concerning blood products
    A. Fresh frozen plasma (FFP) should be ABO compatible with the recipient
    B. Human albumin solution (HAS) has 20% of the coagulation properties of FFP
    C. FFP contains fibrinogen
    D. Cryoprecipitate contains factor VIII
    E. FFP should be stored at –4°C

11. FFTTT

Cortisol is produced in the adrenal cortex and increases gluconeogenesis as well as the effects mentioned in the question. It has no effect on fatty acid metabolism.

12. TTFTT

The Lack system is a coaxial version of a Mapleson A in which the large inner tube carries exhaled gas. In a Mapleson A the fresh gas is added to the circuit at the common gas outlet. The Bain system is a coaxial Mapleson D. In the Bain, the fresh gas flow is carried in the narrow inner tube.

13. TTTTT

You must know this! In order, the CVP waveform consists of the a wave, the c wave, the x descent, the v wave and the y descent. The a wave is due to atrial contraction. The c wave is due to bulging of the closed tricuspid valve into the right atrium during isovolumetric ventricular contraction. The x descent reflects the fall in right ventricular pressure when the pulmonary valve opens. The v wave occurs as the tricuspid valve opens at the end of isovolumetric ventricular relaxation at the beginning of diastole. The y descent reflects rapid emptying of the right atrium into the right ventricle after the tricuspid valve has opened.

14. TFTTF

HAS has no significant clotting activity, as it is prepared from plasma that has not been snap frozen to preserve coagulation factors. FFP contains all clotting factors but their concentration is at most that of the normal circulation. Cryoprecipitate on the other hand contains 50% of the fibrinogen, fibronectin and factor VIII of a single blood donation in a volume of 20 ml. FFP should be stored at $-40°C$.

15. Regarding the composition of body fluids
  A. The intracellular fluid volume comprises 60% of the total body water (TBW)
  B. TBW as a percentage of body weight is less in men than in women
  C. The osmolality of plasma is 290 mosmol/kg
  D. As a percentage of body weight, the TBW is greater in the neonate than the adult
  E. The concentration of sodium in the intracellular fluid is 30 mmol/l

16. Ephedrine
  A. Ephedrine is a pure α agonist
  B. 25% of a dose of ephedrine is excreted unchanged in the urine
  C. Ephedrine has no effect on bronchioles
  D. Ephedrine relaxes uterine smooth muscle
  E. The intravenous preparation of ephedrine contains 3 mg/ml

17. Regarding humidification
  A. The latent heat of vaporization of water at room temperature is 2.43 kJ/kg
  B. Doubling the temperature of humidified gas doubles the relative humidity
  C. The absolute humidity of fully saturated air at 37°C is 44 g/m^3
  D. 15% of the total basal heat loss during anaesthesia is due to warming and humidifying inspiratory gases
  E. Water droplets produced by nebulizers should be greater than 5 μm in diameter

15. TFTTF
Adipose tissue contains relatively little water. As there is a higher proportion of adipose tissue in females the TBW is less in women than in men. The plasma osmolality predominantly depends on the plasma concentrations of sodium, chloride, urea and glucose. Therefore plasma osmolality is 2 × [Na] + [glucose] + [urea] = 2 × 140 + 5 + 5 = 290 mosmol/kg. The concentration of sodium in the intracellular fluid is 10 mmol/l while in the plasma it is 145 mmol/l.

16. FFFTF
Ephedrine is an α and β agonist. Up to 99% is eliminated unchanged in the urine. Ephedrine causes bronchodilation and relaxes uterine smooth muscle. In the ampoule the concentration of ephedrine is 30 mg/ml.

17. FFTTF
The latent heat of vaporization of water at room temperature is 2.43 MJ/kg. Increasing temperature reduces the relative humidity. For example, fully saturated air at 20°C contains 17 g/m³ water vapour. If the air is then heated to 37°C the mass of water vapour or absolute humidity in a given volume of air is the same. However the mass of water that could be present in the air at 37°C if it were fully saturated is 44 g/m³. Remember that relative humidity is the mass of water actually present divided by the mass of water that would be required to saturate. In this example therefore the relative humidity of water in air heated to 37°C is 17/44 or 39%. Water droplets greater than 5 μm are deposited in the trachea and do not reach the alveolus. The ideal size is 1 μm.

18. Regarding temperature
   A. The resistance of a platinum wire rises as its temperature falls
   B. The change in electrical resistance of a metal with change in temperature is known as the Seebeck effect
   C. A thermistor generates a current
   D. A thermocouple is made of a metal oxide
   E. The electrical resistance in a thermocouple is exponentially related to the temperature of the object being measured

19. Concerning diuretics
   A. Bendrofluazide mainly acts on the proximal convoluted tubule
   B. Thiazide diuretics cause hypercalcaemia
   C. Potassium loss is greater with loop diuretics than with thiazide diuretics
   D. Furosemide inhibits the reabsorption of chloride ions in the thick ascending loop of Henle
   E. Thiazides reduce the plasma concentration of lithium in patients receiving lithium treatment

20. Cerebrospinal fluid (CSF)
   A. The normal concentration of glucose in the CSF is 4.8 mmol/l
   B. The volume of the CSF is 300 ml
   C. CSF is produced by the arachnoid villi
   D. CSF is produced at a rate of 600 ml/24 h
   E. The protein content of CSF is 0.3 g/l

18. FFFFF

The electrical resistance in a platinum wire rises in a linear fashion with increasing temperature. A thermistor is made of a metal oxide and requires a battery to produce a current through it. The resistance of a thermistor falls exponentially with rising temperature. A thermocouple is made of two metals such as copper and constantan. At the junction of two different metals, an electrical current is generated. This is the Seebeck effect. The size of the current is proportional to the temperature of the junction compared to a reference junction held at a constant temperature and rises in a linear fashion with the temperature.

19. FTFTF

It is important to know about diuretics. Half of one of the authors' pharmacology viva was about diuretics. Luckily he knew about them, as the other half of the viva was a disaster! Carbonic anhydrase inhibitors, e.g. acetazolamide, act on the proximal convoluted tubule. Bendrofluazide acts on the cortical diluting segment just proximal to the distal convoluted tubule by inhibiting active sodium and chloride reabsorption. As a result, the amount of sodium reaching the distal convoluted tubule is increased, more so than with loop diuretics, so that potassium loss occurs to a greater degree. The side effects of thiazides include metabolic alkalosis, hyperglycaemia, calcaemia, lipidaemia and uricaemia, and hypovolaemia, kalaemia and natraemia. By reducing sodium reabsorption, thiazides may increase lithium reabsorption and precipitate toxicity in patients receiving lithium treatment.

20. TFFTT

The majority of the CSF is produced by the choroid plexus. Some (30%) is produced by the endothelium of cerebral capillaries. The volume of CSF is 150 ml. The glucose concentration (non-fasting) in plasma and CSF is 8 mmol/l and 4.8 mmol/l, respectively.

21. Regarding red blood cells
  A. Erythropoietin (EPO) is mainly produced in the liver
  B. Acidosis increases the affinity of haemoglobin for oxygen
  C. Fetal haemoglobin consists of two α and two γ chains
  D. The typical haemoglobin concentration in a 1 year old child is 16 g/dl
  E. 2,3–diphosphoglycerate (2,3–DPG) is found in red blood cell mitochondria

22. Regarding electrical resistance
  A. The Wheatstone bridge circuit consists of four resistors
  B. The heat generated when a current flows through a resistance is proportional to the square of the resistance
  C. The ohm is that resistance which will allow the flow of 1.63×10^7 electrons to flow past a point in 1 s
  D. The resistance of a wire increases as it is stretched
  E. The impedance of antistatic theatre shoes should be between 10 and 50 kΩ

23. The following can be measured directly with a spirometer
  A. Vital capacity (VC)
  B. Inspiratory reserve volume (IRV)
  C. Residual volume (RV)
  D. Functional residual capacity (FRC)
  E. Tidal volume (TV)

21. **FFTFF**
    The kidney is the main producer of the glycoprotein EPO, although some is formed in the liver. Deoxyhaemoglobin is a better proton acceptor than oxyhaemoglobin (Haldane effect). Therefore, acidosis favours the formation of deoxyhaemoglobin. In other words, oxyhaemoglobin more readily gives up oxygen in acidic conditions, i.e. its affinity for oxygen decreases. Acidosis therefore shifts the oxygen dissociation curve to the right (Bohr effect). Normal values (g/dl) for haemoglobin concentration are 16–20 for the newborn, 10–12 for a 6 month old infant, and 10.5–13 for a 1 year old. 2,3–DPG is bound to haemoglobin and reduces the oxygen affinity of haemoglobin 26-fold.

22. **TFFTF**
    Look up the Wheatstone bridge circuit in a textbook. It crops up in vivas as well as MCQs and many bits of monitoring equipment, e.g. pressure transducers. As $P = I^2R$ (where P is power, or heat generated in watts, and I is the current flowing through a resistance R), heat production is proportional to the square of the current. This principle is used in diathermy. Answer C above is rubbish. The ohm is that resistance which will allow 1 ampere of current to flow under the influence of a potential of 1 volt. Antistatic shoes should have an impedance of 75 kΩ to 10 MΩ. It should be high enough to prevent mains-related electric shock by reducing the size of current which can flow through the body ($I = V/R$), while allowing static charge to flow to earth to prevent microshock.

23. **TTFFT**
    RV and FRC can be deduced from spirometry but cannot be measured directly using this method. The body plethysmograph and helium dilution methods are used to determine FRC and RV directly.

24. The following act on cholinergic receptors
A. Suxamethonium
B. Pilocarpine
C. Trimetaphan
D. Procyclidine
E. Chlorpromazine

25. Regarding gases
A. 1380 l of oxygen are available from a full 10 l oxygen cylinder
B. The Poynting effect describes the working of the cryoprobe
C. Doubling the temperature of a constant volume of gas from 100°C to 200°C doubles the pressure it exerts
D. 32 g of oxygen contains the same number of molecules as 1 g of hydrogen
E. 44 g of nitrous oxide occupies 22.4 l at 0°C and 101.3 kPa

26. The following are monoamine oxidase inhibitors (MAOIs)
A. Phenelzine
B. Imipramine
C. Lithium
D. Fluoxetine
E. Sertraline

24. TTTTT
Pilocarpine is a muscarinic agonist used to constrict the pupil in glaucoma. Trimetaphan antagonizes nicotinic receptors in autonomic ganglia causing hypotension. Procyclidine is a centrally acting muscarinic antagonist used in the treatment of Parkinson's disease. Chlorpromazine is a phenothiazine antipsychotic drug that has quite marked antimuscarinic side effects such as dry mouth and blurred vision.

25. TFFFT
Question A relates to Boyle's law. The gauge pressure of a full oxygen cylinder is 13 700 kPa while the absolute pressure is 13 800 kPa. 13 800 kPa × 10 l = 100 kPa × 1380 l. As gas expands on leaving the tip of a cryoprobe the temperature falls. This is an example of an adiabatic change, i.e. a change in volume of a gas without the transfer of heat to or from it. The Poynting effect describes how a nitrous oxide/oxygen mixture is gaseous at a temperature and pressure at which nitrous oxide on its own would be a liquid. Question C refers to the third gas law. Doubling the *absolute* temperature, i.e. from 373 K (100°C) to 746 K (473°C) of a constant volume of gas doubles the pressure. 32 g of oxygen contains the same number of molecules as 2 g of hydrogen, i.e. 1 mole (Avagadro's hypothesis). 1 mole of nitrous oxide (44 g) occupies 22.4 l at standard temperature and pressure (s.t.p.) (273 K and 101.3 kPa).

26. TFFFF
Imipramine is a tricyclic antidepressant. Fluoxetine (Prozac) and sertraline (Lustral) are selective serotonin re-uptake inhibitors (SSRIs) as is paroxetine (Seroxat).

27. During turbulent flow of a fluid in a tube
A. Flow rate is inversely proportional to the viscosity of the fluid
B. Flow rate is inversely proportional to the density of the fluid
C. The pressure difference along the tube must be increased by a factor of four to double the flow
D. The flow rate is directly proportional to the radius of the tube
E. The length of the tube has no effect on the flow rate of fluid through it

28. Regarding pure competitive antagonist drugs
A. The efficacy of a pure antagonist is less than 0.5 but greater than 0
B. Pure antagonist drugs cause a parallel shift to the right of the log-dose-response curve of the agonist
C. The maximal response of a pure agonist is reduced by 25% by a pure antagonist
D. The affinity of an antagonist is inversely proportional to the dissociation constant
E. The efficacy of an agonist is reduced by the addition of an antagonist

29. Concerning the fetal circulation
A. The PaO_2 is highest in the umbilical artery
B. The PaO_2 is 4 kPa in the umbilical vein
C. The ductus venosus connects the pulmonary artery to the aorta
D. The fetal oxygen dissociation curve is shifted to the left compared to the adult
E. The lungs receive 100% of the total cardiac output

27. FTTFF

In turbulent flow, Q is proportional to $r^2\sqrt{P/l\rho}$, where Q is the flow rate, r is the radius of the tube, l is the length of the tube, P is the pressure across the tube and ρ is the density of the fluid. The flow rate is therefore proportional to the radius squared. In laminar flow, the flow rate is directly proportional to the pressure difference along the tube. In turbulent conditions, however, the rate of flow is proportional to the square root of the pressure difference. Therefore to double the flow, the pressure needs to be quadrupled.

28. FTFTF

The efficacy of a pure antagonist is 0, i.e. it has no effect. The maximal response of an agonist is not reduced as a pure competitive antagonist can always be completely overcome by increasing the concentration of the agonist. The maximal response of the agonist in the presence of an antagonist therefore is still 100% although its dose will have to be increased. The efficacy of an agonist is 1 and is unaffected by the presence of an antagonist.

29. FTFTF

The PaO_2 is highest in the umbilical vein. The umbilical vein empties into the inferior vena cava via the ductus venosus. The ductus arteriosus connects the pulmonary artery to the aorta. The fetal lungs only receive 15% of the total cardiac output.

30. The following coagulation factors are involved in the intrinsic coagulation pathway
   A. Factor XII
   B. Factor XI
   C. Factor II
   D. Factor VIII
   E. Factor VII

31. Concerning solubility
   A. As a liquid is warmed more gas is dissolved in it
   B. Nitrous oxide is less soluble in water than nitrogen
   C. The Bunsen solubility coefficient is the volume of gas which dissolves in one unit volume of the liquid at the temperature concerned
   D. 0.39 l of nitrous oxide will dissolve in 1 l of blood at 37°C at atmospheric pressure
   E. The oil/gas partition coefficient of nitrous oxide is 0.47

32. Regarding the cardiac muscle action potential
   A. The resting membrane potential is –90 mV
   B. Phase 1 is rapid depolarization
   C. Phase 2 is due to calcium influx
   D. Cardiac muscle cells depolarize to +70 mV
   E. Phase 3 is ATP-ase dependent

30. TTTTF
Although there are several different coagulation models, you have to know the classical one as it is very easy to ask MCQs about.

31. FFFFF
As a liquid is warmed less gas dissolves in it, e.g. as water is heated bubbles appear. Nitrous oxide is much more soluble than nitrogen. At 37°C, 1 l of water will dissolve 0.014 l of nitrogen and 0.39 l of nitrous oxide. The blood gas partition coefficient of nitrous oxide is 0.47. Therefore 0.47 l of nitrous oxide will be dissolved in 1 l of blood at 37°C. The oil/gas partition coefficient of nitrous oxide is 1.4. The Bunsen solubility coefficient is corrected to s.t.p. The definition in question C is for the Ostwald solubility coefficient.

32. TFTFF
Phase 0 is rapid depolarization to +20 mV and is due to opening of the fast sodium channels with influx of sodium into the cell. Phase 1 is early rapid repolarization and is due to potassium efflux. Phase 2 is the plateau phase of repolarization in which the efflux of potassium is balanced by the influx of calcium. Phase 3 is due to increased potassium efflux and results in rapid depolarization. It is not energy dependent. Phase 4, however, is dependent on ATPase pumps that exchange intracellular calcium and sodium for potassium.

33. **The following can be used to measure anaesthetic vapour concentrations**
    A. Infrared analysers
    B. Riken gas analysers
    C. Dräger Narkotest
    D. Hook and Tucker analyser
    E. Parlour and Adams analyser

34. **Regarding the ECG**
    A. The normal QRS complex has a duration <0.2 s
    B. The Q–T interval is measured from the end of the Q wave to the beginning of the T wave
    C. Hypermagnesaemia prolongs A–V conduction time
    D. Lead III of the ECG is recorded between the left arm and the left foot
    E. An R–R interval of five large squares on an ECG recorded with a paper speed of 25 mm/s occurs when the heart rate is 100 beats/min

35. **Regarding barbiturates**
    A. Methohexitone has a hydrogen atom at position 4 of the barbiturate ring
    B. Thiopentone has a methyl group at position 2 of the barbiturate ring
    C. In thiopentone the alkyl groups at position 5 of the barbiturate ring contain double bonds
    D. Barbituric acid has hypnotic properties
    E. Thiopentone has a sulphur atom at position 1 of the barbiturate ring

33. TTTTF

All anaesthetic vapours absorb infrared light. The Riken gas analyser measures the difference between the refractive index of light in clean air and air containing the gas being measured. The Dräger Narkotest measures the change in the elasticity of rubber when anaesthetics dissolve in it. Halothane absorbs ultraviolet light with a maximum absorption in the region of 200 nm. The Hook and Tucker meter depends on the ability of halothane to absorb ultraviolet light. Ray Parlour and Tony Adams are the cornerstones of Arsenal Football Club, and although they have done many miraculous things on the pitch, they have not yet invented an anaesthetic gas analyser. But then again Hook and Tucker can't play football.

34. FFTTF

The duration of the normal QRS complex is < 0.12 s (three small squares). The normal PR interval is < 0.2 s (five small squares). The Q–T interval is measured from the beginning of the Q wave to the end of the T wave. The normal recording speed of the ECG is 25 mm/s. At this speed, each large square, which is 5 mm wide, represents 0.2 s. Therefore, five large squares are 1 s and correspond to a heart rate of 60 beats/min. To work out the heart rate quickly, divide 300 by the number of large squares that make up the R–R interval.

35. FFFFF

You have to know the structure of barbiturates. Methohexitone and thiopentone have an oxygen atom at position 4 of the barbiturate ring. At position 1 thiopentone has a hydrogen atom while methohexitone has a methyl group. At position 2 thiopentone has a sulphur atom while methohexitone has an oxygen atom. The alkyl group at position 5 of the barbiturate ring only contains double bonds in methohexitone. Barbituric acid has no hypnotic effect. It is the addition of alkyl groups to the ring, which confers hypnotic properties.

36. Regarding neuromuscular monitoring
  A. The appearance of one twitch following a train of four (TOF) stimulus corresponds to 90% receptor blockade
  B. Following a TOF stimulus, the ratio between the height of the fourth and first twitches should be greater than 50% for adequate respiratory function
  C. A post tetanic twitch count of 15 is equivalent to two twitches of a TOF
  D. The fourth twitch of a TOF appears when less than 75% of receptors are blocked
  E. Tetanic fade occurs in patients who have received mivacurium

37. Midazolam
  A. Midazolam is water soluble but has a very low lipid solubility
  B. Midazolam causes muscle relaxation by a direct action on myofibrils
  C. There are three types of benzodiazepine receptor
  D. The elimination half-lives of midazolam and diazepam are similar
  E. Midazolam is 95% bound to albumin in the plasma

38. Sources of error in oximetry
  A. The presence of methaemoglobin results in a reading for oxygen saturation of 85%
  B. HbS causes under reading of the true oxygen saturation
  C. Carboxyhaemoglobin results in over estimation of the oxygen saturation
  D. Methylene blue reduces oximeter readings by up to 65%
  E. Anaemia has no effect on oxygen saturation readings

36. TFTTT
For adequate respiratory function the T4/T1 ratio should be greater than 70%. A post tetanic twitch count of less than five indicates profound neuromuscular block whereas a count of 15 or more means that reversal of the block will succeed. Tetanic fade occurs following competitive neuromuscular blockade.

37. FFTFT
All the benzodiazepines are highly lipid soluble, midazolam being the most. However, apart from midazolam they are insoluble in water. Midazolam causes muscle relaxation by a direct effect on the dorsal horn of the spinal cord. Three types of benzodiazepine receptor are found in the brain and spinal cord and are responsible for the various effects of these drugs, e.g. ω_1 is responsible for sedation, while ω_2 is responsible for the anticonvulsant effects. The half-lives of midazolam and diazepam are 5 h and 30 h, respectively.

38. TFTTF
The pulse oximeter measures the absorbance of light at two wavelengths, 660 nm and 940 nm. Methaemoglobin absorbs more light than both oxy- and deoxyhaemoglobin at 940 nm and has a similar absorbance to deoxyhacmoglobin at 660 nm. Therefore, at both low and high oxygen saturations, the oximeter reading will be about 85%. Carboxyhaemoglobin has no absorbance at 940 nm but simulates oxyhaemoglobin at 660 nm, which leads to over estimation of the true saturation. HbS has no effect on oximeter readings. As well as methylene blue, dark nail polishes can interfere with oximeter readings. As haemoglobin concentration falls there is a tendency to underestimate the true oxygen saturation.

39. Halothane and enflurane
  A. Halothane has a MAC of 1.68
  B. Halothane should not be used within 6 months of a previous administration
  C. Halothane is 1–bromo-1–chloro-2,2,2–trifluoro-ethane
  D. Carbon monoxide may be produced when enflurane is used with soda lime
  E. Fluoride ion production is greater in the obese patient

40. Pulmonary vascular resistance is increased by
  A. Hypoxia
  B. Hypercarbia
  C. Histamine
  D. 5–HT
  E. Isoprenaline

41. Regarding alfentanil
  A. Alfentanil is more protein bound than morphine
  B. Alfentanil has a higher volume of distribution than fentanyl
  C. Alfentanil has a higher clearance than fentanyl
  D. Alfentanil is predominantly unionized at physiological pH
  E. Alfentanil is an OP_3 receptor agonist

39. FFTTT
The MAC of halothane is 0.75 while the MAC of enflurane is 1.68. The Committee on the Safety of Medicine (CSM) recommends that halothane should not be used within 3 months of a previous administration or if there was unexplained jaundice or fever within a week of a previous halothane anaesthetic. Exhausted soda lime is dry. When the three structurally related vapours isoflurane, desflurane or enflurane are used with dry (exhausted) soda lime, carbon monoxide can be produced. The metabolism of enflurane yields fluoride ions, the amount of which is greater in the obese, particularly the morbidly obese patient.

40. TTTTF
As well as those mentioned in the question, α-sympathomimetics increase pulmonary vascular resistance. Pulmonary vascular resistance is reduced by isoprenaline, β-sympathomimetics, acetylcholine, aminophylline and sodium nitroprusside.

41. TFFTT
Morphine is only 35% protein bound compared to alfentanil, which is 92% bound to protein. The volume of distribution of alfentanil (0.8 l/kg) is much less than that of fentanyl (4 l/kg) because alfentanil is less lipid soluble than fentanyl. Alfentanil has a lower clearance than fentanyl (6 ml/kg/min vs 13 ml/kg/min). Despite this, the terminal half-life of alfentanil is shorter than fentanyl's as the volume of distribution is so much less. In fact, the clearance of alfentanil is significantly less than all the other commonly used opioids. Alfentanil has a pKa of 6.5 so that it is 89% unionized at physiological pH compared to fentanyl, which has a pKa of 8.4 and is only 9% unionized at the same pH. The rapid speed of onset is attributable to the high percentage of alfentanil that exists in the plasma in the unionized form as well as to its lipophilicity. Alfentanil is an OP_3 (μ) receptor agonist.

42. The following antiemetics are 5–HT$_3$ receptor antagonists
  A. Hyoscine
  B. Droperidol
  C. Prochlorperazine
  D. Ondansetron
  E. Metoclopramide

43. Regarding pH
  A. A 1 molar solution of hydrochloric acid (HCl) has a pH of 0
  B. pH = log$_{10}$ [H$^+$]
  C. The pH electrode contains two metal electrodes
  D. A potential difference dependent upon the pH of the sample develops between the measuring and reference electrodes of a pH meter
  E. The pH electrode does not require a battery

44. Regarding the nerve supply to the body
  A. The knee jerk reflex involves L1–L2
  B. Sensory supply to the umbilical area is from T12
  C. The hand receives innervation from C6, C7 and C8
  D. Elbow flexion is supplied by C5 and C6
  E. The skin over the anterior aspect of the upper thigh is mainly supplied by L2

45. Concerning vaporizers
  A. The EMO vaporizer is temperature compensated
  B. The EMO vaporizer is used with ether
  C. The Oxford Miniature Vaporizer (OMV) is only used with halothane
  D. The Goldman vaporizer is a draw-over vaporizer
  E. The OMV uses a bimetallic strip for temperature compensation

42. FTFTT
Ondansetron is a pure $5HT_3$ receptor antagonist. Other pure $5HT_3$ receptor antagonists are granisetron and tropisetron, while droperidol and chlorpromazine have some anti-$5HT_3$ properties. Hyoscine is anti-muscarinic and prochlorperazine is anti-dopaminergic.

43. TFTTT
pH = $-\log_{10}$ [H$^+$]. The concentration of hydrogen ions, [H$^+$], in a 1 molar solution of HCl is 1 mmol/l. Therefore, pH = $-\log_{10}1$ = 0. If the solution was 0.1 molar, the pH would be $-\log_{10}$ [0.1] = 1. Another way of looking at this is as follows: [H$^+$] = 10^{-p} so that if [H$^+$] is 0.01 mmol/l as in a 0.01 molar solution of HCl, then pH is 2 as 10^{-2} = 0.01. The pH electrode has silver/silver chloride and mercury/mercury chloride electrodes.

44. FFTTT
Nerves from L3–L4 mediate the knee jerk reflex. Sensory supply to the umbilical area is from T10.

45. TTFTF
The EMO ether inhaler is temperature compensated by means of an ether bellows which expands and contracts depending on the temperature, allowing different amounts of carrier gas into the vaporization chamber. There is also a water heat sink. The OMV has detachable scales so that it can be used with different anaesthetics. It is not temperature compensated but does have a water and anti-freeze heat sink.

46. Adrenaline
  A. Is the neurotransmitter at the sympathetic ganglia
  B. Constitutes the main secretion from adrenergic neurones
  C. Is blocked by trimetaphan
  D. Causes dilatation of the pupil
  E. 200 ml of 1: 200 000 contains 1 mg adrenaline

47. Aspirin
  A. Aspirin has a p*K*a of 7.2
  B. Aspirin mediates its analgesic effects by inhibition of cyclo-oxygenase-2 (COX-2)
  C. Aspirin induced asthma affects between 10 and 20% of adults with asthma
  D. Aspirin inhibits the production of leukotrienes from arachidonic acid
  E. Aspirin overdose causes a respiratory alkalosis

48. Regarding saturated vapour pressure (SVP)
  A. SVP is dependent on the ambient temperature
  B. A liquid boils when its SVP equals atmospheric pressure
  C. At high altitude water will boil at a lower temperature than at sea level
  D. The higher the SVP of a liquid, the higher the temperature at which it boils
  E. The SVP of isoflurane at an atmospheric pressure of 200 kPa is half that at 100 kPa

46. FFFTT
Acetylcholine is the neurotransmitter in sympathetic ganglia and trimetaphan is a ganglion blocker. 90% of the secretion from adrenergic nerves is noradrenaline. 1:1000 adrenaline contains 1 mg/ml, while 1:100 000 contains 1 mg in 100 ml.

47. FTTFT
Aspirin is a weak acid with a pKa of 3.5. COX-2 is responsible for the production of prostaglandins from arachidonic acid which mediate the effects of inflammation, while COX-1 produces prostaglandins which are involved in the maintenance of renal blood flow, platelet function and gastric mucosal protection. COX-2 inhibition is therapeutic whereas COX-1 inhibition causes side effects. Diclofenac and indomethacin, but not aspirin, inhibit lipoxygenase, which produces leukotrienes, one of which, LTB4, is produced during inflammation. Aspirin overdose can cause both a respiratory acidosis, by depression of the respiratory centre, or a respiratory alkalosis by causing hyperventilation due to either increased CO_2 production or a direct stimulatory effect on the respiratory centre. Usually there is also a metabolic acidosis. Respiratory alkalosis is rare in children, as hyperventilation is unusual.

48. TTTFF
SVP is only dependent on ambient temperature. As temperature rises, the SVP rises. When the SVP of a liquid equals atmospheric pressure it will boil. If the ambient pressure falls, e.g. up a mountain, the liquid will boil at a lower temperature. The closer the SVP is to atmospheric pressure, the more volatile it is said to be, as it will boil at a lower temperature (think of desflurane). As SVP is independent of ambient pressure, the SVP of isoflurane is the same at 200 kPa as it is at 100 kPa as long as the temperature is the same.

49. Regarding units of measurement
A. The pascal is the pressure exerted by a force of 1 N/m^2
B. The SI unit of temperature is the centigrade
C. $1 \mu g = 10^{-6} g$
D. The SI unit of mass is the gram
E. A force of 1 N is required to accelerate a mass of 1 kg at 1 m/s^2

50. The following increase gastric acid production
A. β receptor stimulation
B. Gastrin
C. Histamine
D. Prostaglandin E_1
E. Intrinsic factor

51. Regarding the cardiac cycle in a normal adult
A. The dicrotic notch results from closure of the aortic valve
B. The aortic valve opens when the ventricular systolic pressure reaches mean arterial pressure
C. Ventricular end diastolic volume is 120 ml
D. Coronary artery perfusion is greatest at the beginning of ventricular systole
E. The majority of ventricular filling results from atrial contraction

52. Propofol
A. Is 98% protein bound in plasma
B. Is an anticonvulsant
C. Reduces the duration of the convulsion following ECT
D. Is insoluble in water
E. Is conjugated in the liver

49. TFTFT
The SI units of temperature and mass are the kelvin and kilogram, respectively.

50. FTTFF
Histamine, acetylcholine and gastrin stimulate gastric acid secretion. Prostaglandin E_2 inhibits acid production. Intrinsic factor is needed for the absorption of vitamin B_{12}.

51. FFTFF
The dicrotic notch on the arterial waveform is due to elastic recoil of the aorta. The aortic valve opens when the ventricular pressure reaches diastolic pressure and marks the end of isovolumetric ventricular contraction. Coronary artery perfusion mainly occurs during ventricular diastole. Seventy-five percent of ventricular filling occurs in the first two thirds of diastole, particularly early diastole when the mitral or tricuspid valves have opened following isovolumetric relaxation of the ventricle. During the last third of diastole, atrial contraction accounts for 25% of the total ventricular filling.

52. TTTFT
Propofol is minimally soluble in water. It is an anticonvulsant and is used to treat status epilepticus. Propofol is conjugated in the liver with glucuronide to make it water soluble.

53. Regarding the elimination of drugs from the blood
  A. Clearance = dose/AUC (where AUC is area under the curve)
  B. Phenytoin exhibits zero order elimination kinetics
  C. The half-life of a drug is directly proportional to the elimination constant
  D. Clearance is measured in mg/kg/min
  E. Phenytoin exhibits first order elimination kinetics

54. Regarding oxygen failure warning alarms
  A. The whistle lasts for 2 s
  B. The noise level should be 20 dB
  C. The whistle starts when the oxygen supply pressure drops to 260 kPa
  D. The oxygen supply to the failure alarm originates downstream to the rotameters
  E. At an oxygen pressure of 200 kPa the supply of anaesthetic gases is cut off

55. Regarding local anaesthetic drugs
  A. Bupivacaine is significantly more protein bound than ropivacaine
  B. Allergy to procaine is more common than to bupivacaine
  C. Methaemoglobinaemia can occur after using EMLA cream
  D. Local anaesthetic drugs are bound to α_1–acid glycoprotein in the plasma
  E. In the ampoule lidocaine is 99% ionized

53. TTFFT

In zero order kinetics the rate of elimination of a drug is constant irrespective of the plasma concentration of the drug because the elimination pathways are saturated. In first order kinetics the rate of elimination depends on the amount of drug in the plasma. At low plasma concentrations, phenytoin exhibits first order kinetics, while at high concentrations it follows zero-order elimination. The half-life of a drug is inversely proportional to the elimination constant, i.e. the faster a drug is eliminated the shorter its half-life. Clearance is the volume of blood cleared of a drug per unit time and is measured in ml/min.

54. FFTFT

The auditory alarm of the oxygen failure warning device should last for 7 s at a noise level of 60 dB at a distance of 1 m from the anaesthetic machine. The oxygen supply to the alarm arises upstream to the rotameters.

55. FTTTT

Both bupivacaine and ropivacaine are approximately 95% protein bound. Allergy to amide local anaesthetics is rare whereas they are more common with esters. Procaine is metabolized to *para* amino benzoic acid which is allergenic. Methaemoglobinaemia following prilocaine is more common in infants due to immature metabolic processes and can occur after EMLA use. α_1–acid glycoprotein has a high affinity for local anaesthetic in the plasma. The level of α_1–acid glycoprotein in neonates is low, so that the amount of free drug, and consequently the risk of toxicity, is increased. The pKa of all the local anaesthetic drugs is around 8 (lidocaine 7.9). Therefore, in acidic conditions, e.g. inside the nerve cell and in the ampoule, the drug is mainly ionized, whereas in conditions of higher pH, e.g. extracellular fluid, the unionized form predominates.

56. Concerning the diffusion of gases
  A. The rate of diffusion of a gas across a membrane is proportional to the square root of the molecular weight of the gas
  B. Carbon monoxide is used to measure the rate of diffusion across the alveolar capillary membrane
  C. Nitrous oxide diffuses more readily than nitrogen
  D. The rate of diffusion of a gas is proportional to its solubility
  E. Oxygen diffuses more rapidly than carbon dioxide

57. Regarding glucose handling by the kidney
  A. Glucose appears in the urine when the plasma glucose concentration rises above 11 mmol/l
  B. Glucose reabsorption is linked to sodium reabsorption
  C. Glucose is primarily reabsorbed in the distal tubule
  D. Insulin promotes the renal excretion of glucose
  E. Glucose reabsorption occurs passively along its concentration gradient

58. Ketamine
  A. Ketamine solution has a pH of 11
  B. Ketamine is an NMDA receptor agonist
  C. Ketamine increases uterine tone
  D. Ketamine stimulates β_2 receptors causing bronchodilatation
  E. Ketamine is excreted unchanged in the urine and the bile

56. FTTTF
The rate of diffusion of a gas is inversely proportional to the square root of the molecular weight of the gas. This is Graham's law. The rate of diffusion of a gas is also proportional to its solubility. As nitrous oxide is more soluble than nitrogen it diffuses more rapidly. This is why a pneumothorax will expand more rapidly in a patient breathing nitrous oxide, i.e. nitrous oxide will diffuse into the pneumothorax faster than nitrogen will diffuse out. Because carbon dioxide is much more soluble than oxygen it will diffuse a great deal faster. As well as those factors mentioned above, the rate of diffusion is proportional to the tension gradient across and the surface area of the membrane concerned, and is inversely proportional to the membrane's thickness.

57. TTFFF
When the plasma glucose concentration rises above 11 mmol/l, the tubular maximum for glucose reabsorption is exceeded in some nephrons and glucose appears in the urine. Glucose is reabsorbed in the proximal tubule against its concentration gradient along with sodium. Sodium reabsorption is active. Insulin has no effect on glucose reabsorption by the kidney.

58. FFTFF
Ketamine solutions have a pH of between 3.5 and 5.5. Ketamine is an NMDA receptor antagonist. Ketamine increases uterine tone in both the pregnant and non-pregnant uterus. It is also anticholinergic causing bronchodilatation. Ketamine is metabolized in the liver to norketamine that is then hydroxylated and excreted mainly in the bile, although about 20% appears in the urine. Very little is excreted unchanged.

59. Regarding the measurement of oxygen concentration
   A. The Clarke electrode requires a battery
   B. The fuel cell requires a battery
   C. In the fuel cell electrons flow from the lead anode to the gold cathode
   D. The Clarke electrode has a platinum cathode
   E. Oxygen absorbs ultraviolet light

60. Antidiuretic hormone (ADH)
   A. ADH increases the permeability of the proximal tubule to water
   B. ADH increases the permeability of the collecting tubule to urea
   C. The normal urine osmolality is 200–250 mosmol/l
   D. ADH is formed in the posterior pituitary
   E. High plasma osmolarity stimulates the release of ADH

61. Sevoflurane
   A. Sevoflurane is more volatile than enflurane and isoflurane
   B. Sevoflurane causes a tachycardia
   C. Sevoflurane is a bronchodilator
   D. 3–5% of sevoflurane is metabolized in the liver by cytochrome p450
   E. Compound A is produced in higher concentrations when used in a circle system with baralyme than one using soda lime

62. The following increase lower oesophageal sphincter (LOS) tone
   A. Gastrin
   B. Histamine
   C. β blockade
   D. Cholinergic stimulation
   E. Oestrogen

59. TFTTT
The fuel cell produces a current and does not therefore need a battery to work.

60. FTFFT
ADH is formed in the hypothalamus and stored in secretory granules in the posterior pituitary. It is released in response to osmoreceptors that respond to a high plasma osmolarity. ADH increases the permeability of the collecting tubule to water and urea. It has no effect on the proximal tubule. Urea leaves the tubule in the medulla and helps to maintain the high osmolarity in this part of the kidney. Stem C is false for two reasons. Firstly, osmolality is measured in mosmol/kg of solvent whereas osmolarity is measured in mosmol/l of solvent. Secondly, the normal urine osmolality is 300–350 mosmol/kg while for plasma it is 290 mosmol/kg.

61. FFTTT
The SVPs of sevoflurane, enflurane and isoflurane at 20°C are 21.3 kPa, 22.9 kPa and 31.9 kPa respectively. Sevoflurane causes a bradycardia. The higher the temperature within the carbon dioxide absorber the more compound A is formed from sevoflurane. Baralyme reaches a higher temperature than soda lime.

62. TTTTF
As well as the factors mentioned above, dopaminergic inhibition, α stimulation, motilin and prostaglandins F_2 increase LOS tone. Oestrogen reduces LOS tone as do α inhibition, β and dopaminergic stimulation and prostaglandin E_1.

63. The mole
  A. The mole is that quantity containing the same number
     of particles as there are atoms in 1 g of carbon-12
  B. 1 mole of solute dissolved in 22.4 l of solvent at 0°C
     exerts an osmotic pressure of 101.3 kPa
  C. The mole is temperature dependent
  D. Avogadro's number is 6.022×10^{23}
  E. 1 mole of a gas occupies 22.4 l at s.t.p.

64. Regarding opioid drugs
  A. Pethidine is a phenylpiperidine opioid
  B. 10 mg of morphine hydrochloride is contained in 20 mg
     of papaveretum
  C. The bioavailability of oral buprenorphine is 55%
  D. Methadone is a naturally occurring morphine analogue
  E. Remifentanil is chemically related to pethidine

65. Angiotensin
  A. Angiotensin II is formed in the lung
  B. Renin is produced in the juxtaglomerular apparatus of
     the kidney
  C. Angiotensin II stimulates the release of aldosterone
  D. Angiotensin II increases sodium reabsorption by the
     proximal tubule of the kidney
  E. Renin stimulates thirst

63. FTFTT
The mole is the SI unit of quantity. The mole is that quantity containing the same number of particles as there are atoms in 12 g of carbon-12. Stem C is nonsense as the mole is a number and is not dependent on anything. Avogadro's number is the number of atoms in 12 g of carbon-12. By the way, s.t.p. is standard temperature and pressure which is 0°C and 101.3kPa.

64. TFFFT
Papaveretum (Omnopon) contains a mixture of soluble opioids found in opium including morphine (50%), codeine (5%) and papaverine (5%). Prior to reformulation, when it also contained 20% narcotine (noscapine), 20 mg of papaveretum contained 10 mg of morphine hydrochloride. The narcotine was removed, as it is teratogenic in animals, while the amounts of the other opioids were kept as in the original ampoule, so that now 10 mg of morphine hydrochloride is contained in 15.4 mg of papaveretum. 10 mg of morphine hydrochloride is equivalent to 13.3 mg of morphine sulphate. Buprenorphinc has a high first-pass metabolism so its oral bioavailability is only 15%. When given sublingually however, the bioavailability increases to 55% as it is very lipophilic. Methadone is a synthetic morphine analogue. Remifentanil, fentanyl, alfentanil, sufentanil and phenoperidine are all, like pethidine, phenylpiperidines.

65. TTTTF
Renin is released in response to poor renal perfusion and produces angiotensin I from angiotensinogen. Angiotensin-converting enzyme (ACE) forms angiotensin II in the lungs from angiotensin I. As well as the effects mentioned in the question, angiotensin II is a vasoconstrictor, particularly intrarenally. It also stimulates the release of ADH and causes thirst, and inhibits the further release of renin.

66. Concerning intravenous fluid and electrolyte solutions
   A. The pH of normal saline is 7.4
   B. The concentration of calcium ions in 10% calcium gluconate is greater than in 10% calcium chloride
   C. Dextrose 4% saline 0.18% contains 50 mmol/l of sodium
   D. The osmolality of 10% dextrose is double that of 5% dextrose
   E. 8.4% sodium bicarbonate solution contains 1000 mmol/l of sodium

67. The following are class I antiarrhythmic drugs
   A. Flecainide
   B. Diltiazem
   C. Lidocaine
   D. Sotalol
   E. Disopyramide

68. Regarding oxygen
   A. Oxygen has a boiling point of –183°C
   B. The atomic weight of oxygen is 16
   C. Zeolites are used in oxygen concentrators
   D. The temperature inside a vacuum insulated evaporator (VIE) is –235°C
   E. The pressure of the hospital piped oxygen supply is 137 bar

66. FFFTT

The pH of normal saline is 5. All crystalloid solutions are acidic except sodium bicarbonate (8.4% sodium bicarbonate solution has a pH of 8). 10% calcium gluconate contains 0.22 mmol/ml calcium while 10% calcium chloride contains 0.68 mmol/ml. Dextrose 4% saline 0.18% contains 30 mmol/l of sodium. 8.4% sodium bicarbonate solution contains 1000 mmol/l of sodium and 1000 mmol/l of bicarbonate. It is therefore hyperosmolar with an osmolarity of 2000 mosmol/l.

67. TFTFT

Class I drugs are subdivided into three groups. Class IA includes dysopiramide, class IB lidocaine and class IC flecainide. They all act by slowing sodium entry through fast sodium channels and reduce the rate of rise of phase 0 depolarization in non-nodal cardiac cells. Diltiazem is a class IV drug while sotalol has properties of both class II and class III drugs.

68. TTTFF

A zeolite is a hydrous silicate which retains nitrogen from compressed air. Oxygen concentrators produce 90% oxygen from air. The melting point of oxygen is –218°C, therefore at –235°C oxygen would be a solid. The temperature inside a VIE is between –160°C and –180°C. The pressure inside a full oxygen cylinder is 137 bar. In the hospital pipeline the pressure is 4 bar.

69. **Concerning cardiac output**
    A. Cardiac output is proportional to the area under the temperature-time curve when the thermodilution method for measuring cardiac output is used
    B. The Fick principle of measuring cardiac output depends upon the injection of a dye into the patient
    C. In a 70 kg man the normal cardiac index is 3–3.5 l/min
    D. The use of PEEP increases cardiac output
    E. The normal systemic vascular resistance (SVR) is 900–1400 dyne s/cm^5

70. **Regarding Rotameter-type flowmeters**
    A. Gas flow readings are taken from the top of the bobbin
    B. The Rotameter tube is parallel sided
    C. Flow is dependent on the density of the gas at low flow rates
    D. A ball valve controls the gas flow through the Rotameter
    E. Each bobbin is matched to its own particular tube

69. FFFFT

Cardiac output is inversely proportional to the area under the temperature-time curve when using the thermodilution method. The Fick principle states that the amount of a substance taken up by an organ per unit time is equal to the arterio-venous (A–V) difference of that substance multiplied by the blood flow. To measure cardiac output using the Fick principle, oxygen uptake is measured. Therefore, $CO = VO_2/(CaO_2 - CvO_2)$, where CO is cardiac output, VO_2 is oxygen uptake in the lungs in litres per minute and $(CaO_2 - CvO_2)$ is the a–v oxygen difference. The normal cardiac index in a 70 kg man is 3–3.5 l/min/m² (beware of questions where a correct value is given with the wrong units). PEEP reduces venous return, cardiac filling and initial fibre length leading to a fall in contractility and cardiac output.

70. TFFFT

The Rotameter tube is tapered, wider at the top than at the bottom. This allows more accurate measurement at low flow rates. The orifice, i.e. the gap between the bobbin and the tube, at the bottom of the tube is narrow so that flow is laminar, while at the top, the orifice is wide so that flow is turbulent. Therefore, at low flow rates, the height of the bobbin is dependent on the viscosity of the gas, while at high flow rates the density is important. A needle valve controls the flow of gas into the Rotameter. Each tube and bobbin are specific for each other and for the gas that they measure. Another gas cannot be used and if the tube breaks, it must be replaced by a new tube/bobbin combination.

71. Anaemia
   A. The normal haemoglobin concentration in adult females is 13–17 g/dl
   B. The concentration of 2,3–diphosphoglycerate (2,3–DPG) in red blood cells in chronic anaemic patients is decreased
   C. Iron deficiency anaemia is microcytic and normochromic
   D. Patients who are homozygous for HbC suffer severe sickling of red blood cells when the oxygen tension in the blood is low
   E. Hypothyroidism causes a macrocytic anaemia

72. Regarding the Manley ventilator
   A. The Manley ventilator is a constant flow generating ventilator
   B. The pressure generated by the Manley ventilator is adjustable
   C. The Manley ventilator has two bellows
   D. The Manley ventilator is volume controlled
   E. The Manley ventilator is time cycled

73. Pethidine
   A. Oral pethidine undergoes significant first-pass metabolism
   B. Pethidine has cholinergic effects
   C. Pethidine does not cross the placenta and is therefore useful in labour
   D. Pethidine is less lipid soluble than morphine
   E. Pethidine is poorly absorbed from the GI tract

71. FFFFT
The normal haemoglobin concentration in adult males is
13–17 g/dl, while in females it is 12–16 g/dl. The
concentration of 2,3–DPG rises in anaemia, shifting the
oxygen dissociation curve to the right, improving the off
loading of oxygen in the tissues. Iron deficiency anaemia is
microcytic and hypochromic. Patients who are homozygous
for HbC suffer minimally with sickling. Patients with
haemoglobin SC disease (those heterozygous for HbS and
HbC) however, have a mild form of sickle cell disease as the
presence of HbC makes the HbS more likely to sickle.

72. FTTTT
The Manley ventilator generates a constant pressure. The
pressure is dependent on the position of the weight on the
external bellows, which is adjustable and is in the region of
1.5 kPa. This is relatively low compared to the pressure in
the patient's lungs. Therefore changes in the resistance and
compliance of the patient's lungs will affect the flow rate
generated by the ventilator. Consequently, the Manley
ventilator does not generate a constant flow and may not be
able to overcome high resistance, e.g. asthma. The Manley
ventilator has an internal and external bellows. It delivers a
set volume depending on the position of the lever on the
arm of the outer bellows. Inspiratory time, i.e. cycling from
inspiration to expiration, is controlled by the filling of the
internal bellows.

73. TFFFF
Pethidine, in common with the other opioids, is mainly in
the unionized form in the alkaline small intestine and is
therefore well absorbed. However, a significant first-pass
effect in the bowel wall and liver reduces its bioavailability.
Pethidine has anticholinergic effects. Pethidine does cross
the placenta and reaches the fetal circulation. However, as it
does not rely totally on conjugation for its metabolism, a
process poorly developed in neonates, it is used in labour.
Pethidine is more lipid soluble than morphine.

74. The following respiratory changes occur during pregnancy
  A. Closing capacity (CC) is reduced
  B. Functional residual capacity (FRC) is reduced
  C. Dead space is reduced
  D. $PaCO_2$ is reduced
  E. Tidal volume is reduced

75. Calcium
  A. Intracellular calcium is at a higher concentration than extracellular calcium
  B. Plasma calcium is lowered by parathyroid hormone
  C. Uptake of calcium from the gut is decreased by 1,25–dihydroxycholecalciferol
  D. Plasma calcium is raised by calcitonin
  E. Hypercalcaemia may present as abdominal pain

76. The following cause plasma cholinesterase deficiency
  A. Hypothyroidism
  B. Etomidate
  C. Pregnancy
  D. Vancomycin
  E. Hypomagnesaemia

74. FTFTF
FRC is reduced by about 25% at term. This is due to falls of 25% in expiratory reserve volume and 15% in residual volume. CC remains unchanged but is more likely to encroach on a reduced FRC during pregnancy especially in the supine position. Due to the dilation of large airways, dead space increases by 45% during pregnancy. Tidal volume also increases by 45%. $PaCO_2$ falls to 3.7–4.2 kPa by the first trimester due to alveolar hyperventilation.

75. FFFFT
The extracellular calcium concentration is in the order of 2 mmol/l while the intracellular calcium concentration is about 10^{-4} mmol/l. Low plasma calcium stimulates parathyroid hormone release. Parathyroid hormone increases plasma calcium by activating osteoclasts. 1,25–dihydroxycholecalciferol (hydroxylated vitamin D) increases the absorption of calcium from the gut. Calcitonin increases the uptake of calcium into bones so lowering the plasma calcium.

76. TFTFF
The list of factors which cause cholinesterase deficiency needs to be learned as they always ask about them in exams! They include ecothiopate eye drops, ketamine and oral contraceptives. Plasma cholinesterase synthesis is reduced in hypothyroidism and pregnancy. Etomidate reduces cholinesterase activity although the levels are normal.

77. Soda lime
   A. Soda lime contains 94% sodium hydroxide
   B. Soda lime granules should be greater than 10 mesh in size
   C. Desflurane should not be used with circle systems as it decomposes in the presence of soda lime to form toxic products
   D. The reaction between soda lime and carbon dioxide is exothermic
   E. Soda lime has a water content of approximately 15%

78. Ropivacaine
   A. Is presented as a racemic mixture
   B. The clearance of bupivacaine is greater than ropivacaine
   C. Has a p*K*a of 8.1
   D. Is structurally related to bupivacaine
   E. Is more lipid soluble than bupivacaine

79. Regarding electrical safety
   A. An electrical current of 100 mA passing through the body will cause a tingle
   B. The impedance of wet skin is 10 000 ohms
   C. Class II electrical equipment must be double insulated
   D. The leakage current from any equipment which can come in contact with the heart must be less than 500 μA to prevent micro-shock
   E. The inside of rotameters is sprayed with gold croxitine to prevent the build up of static electricity

77. FFFTT

Questions about this subject are popular. Soda lime consists of calcium hydroxide (94%), sodium hydroxide (5%), potassium hydroxide (1%) and silicates to bind the granules together. It also has a water content of 14–19% and contains indicators which change colour when the soda lime is exhausted. Baralyme on the other hand contains calcium hydroxide (80%) and barium octohydrate (20%). The mesh size of the granules should be 4–8. The total volume of the spaces between the granules in the circle canister should be the same as the volume of the granules themselves. Carbon dioxide reacts with soda lime to produce heat. Desflurane can be used safely in circle systems.

78. FFTTF

Bupivacaine is presented as a racemic mixture. Ropivacaine however, is an enantiomer and in solution is present only as S-ropivacaine. The clearance of bupivacaine is 0.58 l/min while for ropivacaine it is 0.73 l/min. Ropivacaine is structurally related to bupivacaine. In fact ropivacaine is the propyl homologue of bupivacaine. Ropivacaine is less lipid soluble than bupivacaine and is much less cardiotoxic. It also preserves motor function to a greater degree.

79. FFTFT

Electrical safety is always a hot topic! Mains electricity passing through the body at 1 mA causes a tingle, 5 mA causes pain, 15 mA is the let go threshold causing muscle spasm, 50 mA causes respiratory arrest, 75 mA causes cardiac arrest, 100 mA causes VF while the heart stops in systole if 5 A passes through the body. The impedance of dry skin is 100 000 ohms whilst that of wet skin is 1000 ohms. As current = potential/impedance and the potential of mains electricity is 240 V, the current flowing through dry skin will only be 2.4 mA while through wet skin it will be 240 mA, enough to cause VF. Class I equipment must be fully earthed, while class III equipment can only work with a low voltage (<24 V). The leakage current from any equipment which can come in contact with the heart must be less than 50 µA to prevent micro-shock.

80. Baroreceptors
   A. Baroreceptors are located in the aortic arch and carotid sinus
   B. The baroreceptor response curve is sigmoid
   C. Aortic baroreceptors are responsible for the Bainbridge reflex
   D. The frequency of neuronal discharge from baroreceptors decreases as blood pressure increases
   E. Carotid sinus baroreceptors are more sensitive to changes in blood pressure than aortic baroreceptors

81. Regarding the minimum alveolar concentration (MAC) of volatile anaesthetic agents
   A. MAC is determined in patients breathing oxygen in 50% nitrous oxide
   B. MAC is increased in acidotic patients
   C. The MAC of nitrous oxide is 75%
   D. MAC is lower in a 6-month-old infant than in a full term neonate
   E. Dexmedetomidine increases MAC

82. The anterior pituitary gland secretes
   A. Growth hormone (GH)
   B. Oxytocin
   C. Prolactin
   D. Thyroid stimulating hormone (TSH)
   E. ACTH

83. Concerning critical temperature
   A. The critical temperature is the temperature at which a substance cannot be liquefied by pressure alone
   B. The critical temperature of nitrous oxide is −34°C
   C. The pseudo-critical temperature is the temperature at which a mixture of gases cannot be liquefied by pressure alone
   D. At room temperature carbon dioxide cylinders contain carbon dioxide vapour
   E. The critical pressure is the pressure required to liquefy a vapour at the critical temperature

80. TTFFT
Although the baroreceptor response curve is sigmoid, it is linear over the mean arterial pressure (MAP) range of 80–180 mmHg. Neuronal discharge increases as MAP increases. However, baroreceptors inhibit the vasomotor centre causing, amongst other responses, vasodilatation. The Bainbridge reflex is tachycardia following a rapid increase in intravascular volume in normovolaemic subjects. It is mediated by type A and B stretch receptors in the atria.

81. FFFFF
MAC is determined in ASA I or II unpremedicated patients breathing the volatile agent in 100% oxygen. MAC is unaffected by acid-base status. The MAC of nitrous oxide is 105%. Neonatal MAC is 15–25% less than that of a 1–6-month-old infant. Dexmedetomidine, like clonidine, is an a_2 agonist which increases the potency of anaesthetic drugs, i.e. reduces MAC.

82. TFTTT
The anterior pituitary gland secretes ACTH, TSH, FSH, LH, GH and prolactin. The posterior pituitary secretes oxytocin and antidiuretic hormone.

83. FFFTT
The critical temperature is the temperature *above* which a substance cannot be liquefied by pressure alone. Below the critical temperature a substance is a vapour whereas above this temperature it is a gas. The critical temperatures of common anaesthetic gases are: nitrous oxide 34°C, oxygen –118°C and carbon dioxide 31°C. At room temperature nitrous oxide and carbon dioxide are vapours while oxygen is a gas. In a mixture of gases, e.g. Entonox, the temperature at which the constituents will separate out is the pseudo-critical temperature. In Entonox cylinders the pseudo-critical temperature is approximately –5.5°C. The critical pressure of oxygen is 50 bar.

84. The following are selective β_1–blockers
   A. Sotalol
   B. Timolol
   C. Metaraminol
   D. Esmolol
   E. Atenolol

85. Heliox
   A. Is supplied in brown cylinders with brown shoulders
   B. The pressure inside a full heliox cylinder is 54 bar
   C. The reduced density results in turbulent flow
   D. Is useful in the treatment of asthma
   E. Is less viscous than air

86. Regarding platelets
   A. Platelets contain von Willebrand's factor
   B. The normal life span of a platelet is 21 days
   C. Platelets produce prostacyclin
   D. Platelets produce thromboxane A_2
   E. von Willebrand's factor is needed for the adhesion of platelets to the endothelium

87. Regarding intravenous cannulae
   A. The flow rate through a 14 standard wire gauge (s.w.g.) cannula is 250–360 ml/min
   B. The outer diameter of a 14 s.w.g. cannula is 2.11 mm
   C. The flow rate through a 16 s.w.g. cannula is 130–220 ml/min
   D. The flow rate through an 18 s.w.g. cannula is 75–120 ml/min
   E. The flow rate through cannulae is tested using normal saline

84. FFFTT
Sotalol and timolol block both β_1 and β_2 receptors. Metaraminol is a sympathomimetic drug with both α and β agonist effects although the former is predominant.

85. FFFFF
Heliox contains 79% helium and 21% oxygen. It is supplied in brown cylinders with brown and white quartered shoulders. The pressure in a full cylinder is 137 bar. Heliox is less dense than air reducing both the tendency to turbulent flow (lowering Reynold's number) and the work of breathing. In lower airway obstruction, air flow remains laminar so that flow is dependent on gas viscosity rather than density. Heliox, being more viscous than air, is not useful in the treatment of asthma.

86. TFFTT
The normal life span of a platelet is 8–14 days. The α granules in platelets contain von Willebrand's factor, which acts as a carrier of factor VIII as well as its main function of being involved with platelet adhesion. Thromboxane A_2, which is formed from arachidonic acid in the platelet, induces platelet aggregation. Prostacyclin, which inhibits platelet aggregation, is formed from arachidonic acid in the endothelial cell.

87. TTTTF
This is a popular topic and can appear in any part of the exam and it is easy to score marks if you know the answers. The flow rate through cannulae is tested using distilled water at a constant temperature of 22°C.

88. Concerning carbon dioxide in the blood
  A. Deoxyhaemoglobin rather than oxyhaemoglobin favours the formation of carbamino compounds
  B. The oxygen dissociation curve is steeper than the carbon dioxide dissociation curve
  C. Arterial blood carries 15 ml carbon dioxide/100 ml of blood
  D. The carbon dioxide dissociation curve is sigmoid
  E. The partial pressure of carbon dioxide in arterial blood is 40 mmHg

89. The following are safe to use in patients with malignant hyperpyrexia (MH)
  A. Neostigmine
  B. Nitrous oxide
  C. Prilocaine
  D. Pethidine
  E. Atracurium

90. The following gases absorb infrared light
  A. Carbon dioxide
  B. Oxygen
  C. Nitrogen
  D. Argon
  E. Helium

91. Regarding Arsenal Football Club
  A. Arsenal were conceived before Preston North End (PNE)
  B. Sir Tom Finney scored 187 league goals for Arsenal
  C. Arsenal have won the double once
  D. Arsenal won the FA Cup Final 1–0 against Huddersfield in 1938
  E. Healey and Mackin are the most potent and dangerous striking partnership in English football at the present time

88. TFFFT
The carbon dioxide dissociation curve is more linear than
the oxygen dissociation curve and does not plateau out. It is
also steeper. For example, 4.7 ml of CO_2 is added to 100 ml
of blood with a change in PCO_2 from 40 to 50 mmHg
compared to only 1.7 ml O_2 being added to 100 ml of blood
for a similar change in PO_2. 100 ml of arterial blood carries
48 ml of carbon dioxide.

89. TTTTT
Known triggers of MH are the volatile anaesthetic drugs
and suxamethonium. All local anaesthetics, opioids and
non-depolarizing muscle relaxants are safe. Atropine,
thiopentone and propofol, as well as nitrous oxide are safe.

90. TFFFF
Only gases made up of two or more different atoms absorb
infrared light, e.g. N_2O, enflurane. Gases containing two
similar atoms, e.g. N_2 and O_2, do not absorb infrared light.

91. FFFFF
Preston North End (PNE) were one of the 12 founding clubs
of the football league in England and played their first game
at Deepdale against Burnley on the 8th September 1888.
PNE won 5–2. Arsenal were elected to the league in 1893 and
it was only after this historic event that football meant
anything at all in England or indeed the rest of the world. Sir
Tom Finney scored 187 league goals for PNE at an average
of a goal every 2.31 games. He is now the president of PNE
(wow!). Arsenal have won the double twice (1970/71 and
1997/98). PNE have only won the double once, although they
have won the league and FA Cup once each on separate
occasions. All these successes occurred way before all but one
(NR) of the authors was born. PNE won the Cup in 1938.
They also finished third that year, 3 points behind Arsenal
who won. A little known and irrelevant fact (NR thinks its
fascinating) is that PNE beat Arsenal 1–0 at Highbury in the
fifth round of the FA cup that year. Healey and Mackin
(who?) play for PNE. Answer E is therefore obviously
nonsense. Please note that PNE is not in the primary syllabus.

MCQ Examination Paper B

1. **Atropine**
   A. Has a weak local anaesthetic effect
   B. Reduces atrial contraction
   C. Is antiemetic
   D. Does not cross the placenta
   E. Causes mydriasis

2. **Regarding the carriage of oxygen in the blood**
   A. *In vitro* 1 g of haemoglobin carries 1.39 ml of oxygen
   B. 0.003 ml of oxygen is dissolved in each 100 ml of blood/mmHg PO_2
   C. The partial pressure of oxygen in mixed venous blood is 6 kPa
   D. The oxygen content of mixed venous blood is 20.1 ml/100 ml of blood
   E. Alkalosis shifts the oxygen dissociation curve to the right

3. **Eutectic mixtures**
   A. Halothane and ether form a eutectic mixture when mixed in a ratio of 2:1
   B. EMLA cream contains 2.5% lidocaine and 2.5% procaine
   C. A eutectic mixture is one whose components cannot be separated by distillation
   D. The boiling point of each liquid in a eutectic mixture is altered by the presence of the other
   E. The melting point of each component in the mixture is lowered

1. **TFTFT**
   Atropine is chemically related to cocaine and has a weak local anaesthetic effect. It increases atrial contractility. Atropine crosses both the placenta and the blood-brain barrier, the latter giving rise to sedation, antiemesis and an anti-Parkinsonian action.

2. **TTTFF**
   In vivo, 1 g of oxygen carries 1.34 ml of oxygen. The reason that this figure is lower than the *in vitro* measurement is that under normal conditions some haemoglobin in the body is in the form of methaemoglobin that cannot combine with oxygen. The amount of oxygen dissolved in 100 ml of plasma in a normal person with a PO_2 of 100 mmHg is 0.3 ml/100 ml. In venous blood this value will be $40 \times 0.003 = 0.12$ ml/100 ml. The oxygen content (ml/100 ml) is ($1.34 \times$ Hb concentration (g/dl) $\times$ oxygen saturation/100) + O_2 dissolved in plasma (ml/100 ml). The oxygen content of venous blood is therefore ($1.34 \times 15 \times 75/100$) + 0.12 = 15.2 ml/100 ml, while for arterial blood it is about 20.1 ml/100 ml. Rightward shift of the oxygen dissociation curve, is caused by acidosis and an increase in temperature, carbon dioxide and the concentration of 2,3–diphosphoglycerate (2,3–DPG).

3. **FFFFT**
   A eutectic mixture is a mixture in which the melting point of each component is lowered. In the case of EMLA (lidocaine 2.5% and prilocaine 2.5%), the local anaesthetics are not in aqueous solution but are in a pure unionized form enhancing absorption into the skin. An azeotrope is a mixture of liquids whose components cannot be separated by distillation as the boiling point of each liquid is altered by the presence of the other so that they become identical (e.g. halothane and ether in a ratio of 2:1).

4. **Low molecular weight heparin (LMWH)**
   A. LMWH predominantly inhibits clotting factor IIa
   B. LMWH markedly reduces platelet aggregation
   C. LMWH has a half-life of 40–90 s
   D. Protamine does not reverse the effects of LMWH
   E. The molecular weight of LMWH ranges from
      3000–8000 daltons

5. **Regarding the action potential in the pacemaker cells of the heart**
   A. Phase 0 is slower in pacemaker cells than in myocardial
      cells
   B. Phase 0 is due to the influx of calcium ions
   C. Phase 4 is due to the leakage of sodium ions into the
      cell
   D. Quinidine reduces the threshold potential in pacemaker
      cells
   E. Phase 2 is shorter in pacemaker cells than in myocardial
      cells

6. **Regarding paramagnetic oxygen analysers**
   A. Oxygen is attracted into a magnetic field
   B. Paramagnetic oxygen analysers consist of nitrogen filled
      dumbbells
   C. Nitric oxide is paramagnetic
   D. Paramagnetic oxygen analysers are inaccurate
   E. Nitrous oxide is paramagnetic

7. **Angiotensin-converting enzyme (ACE) inhibitors**
   A. ACE inhibitors increase sodium retention by the kidney
   B. A dry cough is a common side effect
   C. ACE inhibitors reduce the breakdown of bradykinin
   D. Losartan is an ACE inhibitor
   E. Lisinopril has a longer duration of action than
      enalopril

4. **FFFFT**
   LMWH has its main effect on factor Xa with less activity
   against factor IIa. In comparison, heparin's main effect is on
   factor IIa. As thrombin (factor II) markedly reduces platelet
   aggregation, heparin has a major effect on platelet function.
   LMWH has much less effect on thrombin and so has
   minimal effect on platelet function. LMWH has a half-life of
   40–90 min. Protamine reverses both heparin and LMWH.

5. **TTTFF**
   The slope of phase 0 (rapid depolarization) is less steep in
   pacemaker cells than myocardial cells and is due to calcium
   influx. Sodium influx causes depolarization in myocardial
   cells. Phase 4 is due to sodium leakage which results in a
   steady increase in membrane potential until the threshold
   potential is reached after which rapid depolarization occurs.
   Quinidine and procainamide increase the threshold
   potential, i.e. make it less negative, so that it takes longer for
   phase 4 to reach it. This has the effect of slowing the heart
   rate. Unlike the myocardial action potential, pacemaker
   action potentials have no phase 1 and 2.

6. **TTTFF**
   Most gases, including nitrous oxide, are diamagnetic, i.e.
   repelled by a magnetic field. Oxygen and nitric oxide are
   paramagnetic, i.e. attracted into a magnetic field.
   Paramagnetic analysers are highly accurate.

7. **FTTFT**
   There are two angiotensin II receptors, AT_1 and AT_2.
   Stimulation by angiotensin II of the AT_1 receptor, causes
   vasoconstriction and aldosterone secretion. Aldosterone
   causes the kidney to retain sodium and water. ACE
   inhibitors, therefore, reduce sodium retention by the kidney.
   As ACE also breaks down bradykinin, patients taking ACE
   inhibitors have an increased bradykinin level which causes
   the common side effect of a dry cough. Losartan is an
   angiotensin II receptor antagonist. There is no effect on
   bradykinin breakdown so dry cough is not a problem.
   Lisinopril is a long acting ACE inhibitor.

8. **Regarding pure agonist drugs**
   A. The efficacy is 1
   B. An agonist and antagonist drug with the same dissociation constant have the same affinity
   C. A drug with a dissociation constant of 25 has double the affinity of a drug with a dissociation constant of 50
   D. An agonist always has a higher affinity than a partial agonist
   E. The affinity of a drug is dependent on its efficacy

9. **Insulin**
   A. Insulin is secreted from the α cells in the pancreas
   B. Insulin increases ketone formation
   C. Insulin secretion is inhibited by β-blockers
   A. Thiazide diuretics stimulate insulin secretion
   B. Insulin reduces glycolysis

10. **Regarding humidification**
    A. The unit of absolute humidity is gH_2O/m^3
    B. Heat-moisture exchangers increase dead space
    C. The higher the environmental humidity in theatre, the greater the build up of static electricity
    D. The Swedish nose is 35% efficient
    E. The dew point is the temperature at which air is exactly 50% saturated with water

8. TTTFF
A pure agonist with an efficacy of 1 will combine with a receptor and get the maximum response possible. The affinity of a drug is inversely proportional to the dissociation constant that describes the reaction between the drug and the receptor, i.e. affinity = 1/dissociation constant. The greater the dissociation constant, the more readily the drug dissociates from the receptor and the less the affinity the drug has for the receptor. A drug with a dissociation constant of 25 will have an affinity of 1/25 which is double the affinity of a drug with a dissociation constant of 50 where the affinity equals 1/50. An agonist, a partial agonist and an antagonist can have the same affinity for a receptor if they all have the same dissociation constant. They differ, however, in their efficacies. The agonist will have an effect while the antagonist will have no effect unless an agonist is present in which case it will block it. The affinity of a drug is therefore independent of its efficacy.

9. FFTFF
Insulin is secreted by the pancreatic beta cells. It increases glycolysis, and glycogen, protein, triglycerol and fatty acid synthesis. It reduces glycogenolysis, ketone formation and the breakdown of triglycerides. Hyperglycaemia, beta agonists, acetylcholine and glucagon stimulate insulin secretion. Insulin secretion is inhibited by hypoglycaemia, beta-blockers, alpha agonists, somatostatin, diazoxide, thiazides and volatile anaesthetic agents.

10. TTFFF
The higher the humidity, the less risk of static electricity build up. The Swedish nose is a heat-moisture exchanger and is up to 90% efficient. It increases dead space and resistance to breathing. The dew point is the temperature at which air is 100% saturated with water and condensation occurs and is used in measuring humidity with hygrometers, e.g. Regnault's hygrometer.

11. **Prothrombin time (PT)**
    A. Measuring the PT requires the addition of thromboplastin to the blood sample
    B. PT is prolonged in vitamin K deficiency
    C. PT is prolonged in patients with reduced levels of thrombin
    D. PT measures the intrinsic pathway of the coagulation cascade
    E. PT is used to monitor heparin therapy

12. **Concerning ventilators**
    A. The Manley ventilator is a minute volume divider
    B. The Penlon ventilator can be used with a Bain or circle system
    C. Constant flow generating ventilators have a low internal resistance
    D. Constant flow generators are not suitable for use in asthmatic patients
    E. The Servo ventilator has a driving pressure of 400 kPa

13. **Regarding thiopentone and methohexitone**
    A. Pain on injection is more common with thiopentone
    B. In the powder form, thiopentone but not methohexitone contains 6% anhydrous sodium carbonate
    C. When mixed with water thiopentone has a pH of 11
    D. In the plasma methohexitone is 95% bound to albumin
    E. Urea is formed when thiopentone is metabolized

14. **Regarding skeletal muscle**
    A. The H band represents the area in the sarcomere where the actin and myosin myofilaments overlap
    B. During muscle contraction calcium binds to troponin I
    C. Tropomysin is bound to the actin myofilament
    D. The primary substrate for muscle metabolism is glycogen
    E. Myosin binds to the ryanodine receptor on the actin molecule

11. TTTFF
   PT measures the extrinsic pathway. PT is prolonged in patients with deficiencies of factors VII, X, V and II (thrombin), and in those with hypofibrinogenaemia. Although heparin can prolong PT, the activated partial thromboplastin time is used to monitor heparin therapy. The PT is used to monitor warfarin treatment.

12. TTFFT
   Constant flow generators, such as the Penlon and Servo, have a high internal resistance and therefore a high driving pressure (400 kPa). The resistance and compliance of the patient's lungs therefore, have little effect on the flow rate generated by the ventilator. Constant flow generators are the ventilators of choice for patients with non-compliant lungs or bronchospasm.

13. FFTFT
   Pain on injection is common with methohexitone (80%) but rarely occurs with thiopentone. Both drugs contain 6% anhydrous sodium carbonate. Methohexitone is 50–65% protein-bound compared to 60–80% of thiopentone. Both drugs are mainly bound to albumin. Urea is one of the metabolites formed when the barbiturate ring is cleaved.

14. FFTTF
   The A band is in the centre of the sarcomere and comprises myosin filaments, some of which are overlapped by actin. The H band is found in the centre of the A band where myosin molecules are not overlapped by actin. When an action potential enters a muscle, calcium is released via the ryanodine receptor from the sarcoplasmic reticulum where it is stored. Calcium binds to troponin C, changing the configuration of the troponin I and T subunits, eventually resulting in movement of tropomysin revealing actin binding sites to myosin.

15. Diathermy
A. Diathermy uses a direct electrical current
B. When using monopolar diathermy a plate electrode is required
C. The current density at the plate electrode is high so burns are unlikely
D. In a patient with a cardiac pacemaker bipolar diathermy should be used
E. The diathermy should be earthed to reduce the risk to the patient of electrocution

16. Regarding volatile anaesthetic vapours
A. The structure of desflurane differs from that of enflurane by the replacement of the chlorine atom on position 1 of enflurane by a fluorine atom
B. At 20°C, desflurane has a higher SVP than nitrous oxide
C. The boiling point of isoflurane is lower than the boiling point of sevoflurane
D. The blood gas partition coefficient of sevoflurane is 0.42
E. Sevoflurane is presented with 0.1% thymol

17. The following occur during acclimatization to altitude
A. Hyperventilation
B. Reduced pulmonary artery pressures
C. The oxygen dissociation curve is shifted to the right
D. Greater V/Q mismatch
E. Polycythaemia

15. FTFTF

An alternating current with a frequency of 0.5–1 MHz is used. At these high frequencies, the effects on the heart and skeletal muscle are negligible. Monopolar diathermy requires a plate electrode. This acts as one electrode, whereas the forceps act as the other. If the plate is applied correctly, the current density, i.e. the current per unit area, at the plate is low so that only a small amount of heating occurs. Bipolar diathermy does not require a plate. The electrical current flows down one limb of the forceps and up the other. The dispersal of current into other tissues is negligible and interference with pacemakers is less likely than with monopolar diathermy. If the diathermy is earthed then stray current can take another route to earth through the patient, e.g. via a metal drip stand that the patient may be touching. This could electrocute the patient. By isolating the diathermy from earth, this risk is abolished.

16. FFTFF

Stem A would be true if it referred to the difference between desflurane and isoflurane rather than desflurane and enflurane. At 20°C, the SVP of desflurane and nitrous oxide are 88.5 kPa and 5300 kPa, respectively. Isoflurane boils at 48.5°C (SVP at 20°C is 31.9 kPa) while sevoflurane boils at 58.6°C (SVP at 20°C is 21.3 kPa). The blood gas partition coefficient of sevoflurane is 0.69 while that of desflurane is 0.42. Sevoflurane has no added preservative. 0.1% thymol is added to halothane to protect against decomposition by light.

17. TFTFT

From the alveolar gas equation it follows that reducing $PaCO_2$ by hyperventilating, increases the PaO_2. Due to hypoxic pulmonary vasoconstriction pulmonary artery pressure increases. The increase in pulmonary artery pressure improves the blood flow to the more poorly perfused areas of lung reducing V/Q mismatch. Increased levels of 2,3–DPG shift the oxygen dissociation curve to the right. Other features of acclimatization include an increase in the number of capillaries and mitochondria and an increase in the maximum breathing capacity.

18. Carbon dioxide
   A. Is denser than air
   B. Has a critical temperature of $-31°C$
   C. The pressure in a full carbon dioxide cylinder is 50 bar at room temperature
   D. Is supplied in grey cylinders with black shoulders
   E. Is manufactured by heating magnesium carbonate

19. Regarding adrenergic receptors
   A. α_1 stimulation causes vasoconstriction
   B. Prazocin is an α_1 antagonist
   C. β_1 stimulation causes lipolysis
   D. α_2 stimulation causes platelet aggregation
   E. Phentolamine is an α receptor agonist

20. The following are mediators of peripheral pain
   A. Bradykinin
   B. Histamine
   C. Serotonin
   D. Growth hormone
   E. Prostaglandins

21. Regarding the definitions of physical phenomena
   A. 1 joule is the work done when the point of application of a force of 1 newton moves 1 metre in the direction of the force
   B. The unit of osmolality is osmol/kg
   C. Relative humidity is measured in percent
   D. The tesla is the unit of magnetic field
   E. The poise is the unit of viscosity

22. The following regarding an ampoule of propofol are true
   A. It contains propylene glycol
   B. The pH is 11
   C. It contains 10% soya bean oil
   D. It contains sodium hydroxide
   E. Propofol exists as four stereo isomers

18. TFFFT
Carbon dioxide has a critical temperature of +31°C. It is therefore a vapour at room temperature. It is supplied in grey cylinders with grey shoulders. The pressure inside a full carbon dioxide cylinder at room temperature is 57 bar, while it is 50 bar at 15°C.

19. TTTTF
β_1 stimulation causes lipolysis which increases blood sugar. α_2 stimulation causes platelet aggregation and presynaptically inhibits the release of noradrenaline and acetylcholine. Phentolamine is an α receptor antagonist.

20. TTTFT
These mediators initiate peripheral pain by either altering membrane potentials of pain nerves directly or by activating secondary messengers after stimulating receptors.

21. TTTTT
Osmolality is osmol/kg solvent whereas osmolarity is osmol/l solvent. Absolute humidity is measured in gH_2O/m^3.

22. FFTTF
When asked about the common anaesthetic drugs you must know exactly what you are injecting into a patient. The pH of an ampoule of propofol is 6–8.5. Propofol is dissolved in a mixture of 1.2% egg phosphatide, 10% soya bean oil, 2.25% glycerol, sodium hydroxide and water. Stem E is nonsense. Methohexitone exists as four stereo isomers.

23. The regulation of acid-base balance by the kidney
  A. Phosphate is a renal tubular buffer
  B. Carbonic anhydrase catalyses the reaction $HCO_3^- + H^+$ $\rightarrow H_2CO_3$ in renal tubular cells
  C. Ammonia is synthesized by the kidney from glutamine
  D. Chloride ions in the renal tubules combine with excreted hydrogen ions and thus act as a buffer
  E. The minimum achievable urinary pH is 4.5

24. Remifentanil
  A. Remifentanil has a volume of distribution less than that of alfentanil
  B. Remifentanil is safe to give via the epidural route
  C. Anticholinesterases reduce the metabolism of remifentanil
  D. Remifentanil and fentanyl have similar potencies
  E. Recovery following a remifentanil infusion is dependent on the duration of the infusion

25. Regarding the gas laws
  A. Graham's law relates the size of molecules to their rate of diffusion
  B. Henry's law relates the rate of diffusion of a gas to the surface area of the membrane across which it diffuses
  C. Dalton's law relates to the partial pressure exerted by individual gases in a mixture of gases
  D. Boyle's law describes the relationship between the pressure and volume of a gas at constant temperature
  E. At a constant volume the pressure of a gas is proportional to its temperature

23. TFTFT

Carbonic anhydrase catalyses the reaction $H_2O + CO_2 \rightarrow H_2CO_3$. The minimum pH that the tubules can achieve is 4.5. In other words, the maximum tubular hydrogen ion concentration is $10^{-4.5}$ molar. Without buffering mechanisms therefore, only 1% of the total hydrogen ion production could be excreted by the kidneys. The major tubular buffers are phosphate and ammonia and carry hydrogen in a form other than ionized. This keeps the tubular pH higher than the minimum of 4.5, allowing much more hydrogen to be excreted. Ammonia is formed by the whole renal tubule except for the thin loop of Henle. 60% is formed from glutamine while the remainder comes from other amino acids. When hydrogen combines with chloride ions, hydrochloric acid is formed, which rapidly lowers the pH towards 4.5. Therefore, chloride ions are not buffers, but are in fact excreted combined with ammonium ions that are formed when hydrogen ions are buffered by ammonia.

24. TFFTF

The volume of distribution of remifentanil is 0.35 l/kg. It is the only commonly used opioid whose volume of distribution is less than that of alfentanil (0.8 l/kg). It is metabolized by non-specific plasma and tissue esterases and is not a good substrate for plasma cholinesterase. Therefore, anticholinesterases do not reduce the metabolism or clearance of remifentanil. Remifentanil is formulated in glycine and, therefore, cannot be given epidurally. The low volume of distribution and high clearance (50 ml/kg/min) of remifentanil means that the duration of an infusion has hardly any effect on the recovery time.

25. TFTTT

You should know all the gas laws and the ones concerning solubility (Henry, Ostwald and Bunsen), partial pressure (Dalton) and diffusion (Fick and Graham). Writing them all out here would be boring and make this answer too long. Henry's law by the way relates the amount of gas dissolved in a liquid to the partial pressure of the gas. Stem E is Charles' law.

26. The following are features of a peripheral nerve stimulator
   A. It should produce a sine wave stimulus
   B. The pulse current should be 0.5–5.0 mA when skin electrodes are used
   C. The duration of the stimulus should be 0.2 ms
   D. The train of four (TOF) stimulus consists of four identical stimuli delivered at 4 Hz
   E. A supramaximal stimulus should be avoided as neuronal damage is likely

27. Regarding pKa of local anaesthetic drugs
   A. At a given pH, drugs with a lower pKa will be more unionized than drugs with a higher pKa
   B. Acidosis increases the proportion of ionized drug
   C. pKa is the logarithm to the base 10 ($\log_{10}$) of the dissociation constant
   D. The pKa of bupivacaine is 8.1
   E. At a given pH a higher proportion of bupivacaine will be ionized than lidocaine

28. Concerning blood pressure
   A. The mean arterial pressure (MAP) equals two-thirds of the systolic blood pressure
   B. Pulse pressure equals the systolic minus the diastolic blood pressure
   C. The frequency of baroreceptor discharge increases as blood pressure increases
   D. Atrial natriuretic peptide (ANP) causes hypotension
   E. Bradykinin causes vasoconstriction

29. Regarding gas cylinders
   A. Size G cylinders are larger than size J cylinders
   B. Air cylinders have grey shoulders
   C. The pin index configuration for oxygen is 2 and 5
   D. Entonox cylinders have blue and white quartered shoulders
   E. The pressure in a full nitrous oxide cylinder is 37 bar

26. FFTFF
Peripheral nerve stimulators should produce a square wave stimulus with uniform amplitude lasting for 0.2 ms. A pulse current of 0.5–5.0 mA is adequate when needle electrodes are used. With skin electrodes the current should be supramaximal, i.e. 10–40 mA. This ensures that all muscle fibres are recruited. Supramaximal stimuli do not cause neuronal damage. The frequency of the TOF should be 2 Hz, i.e. 2 per second.

27. TTFTT
$pKa = -\log_{10} Ka$ (where Ka is the dissociation constant). The degree of ionization of a drug at a given pH depends on the Henderson-Hasselbach equation which for basic drugs, such as local anaesthetics states that: $pH = pKa + \log_{10}$ [unionized]/[ionized], where [] is the concentration of drug. Therefore, if the pKa is low then for a given pH the concentration of unionized drug must be higher than the ionized form. Similarly, the lower the pH, the more ionized drug is present. Bupivacaine has a higher pKa than lidocaine (8.1 vs 7.9). Therefore, at a given pH, say 7.4, more bupivacaine will be ionized than lidocaine (85% vs 75%). NB. For acidic drugs the Henderson-Hasselbach equation states that: $pH = pKa + \log_{10}$ [ionized]/[unionized].

28. FTTTF
MAP is approximately equal to the diastolic pressure plus one-third of the pulse pressure. ANP is released when the atria are stretched. Bradykinin causes vasodilatation.

29. FFTTF
The smallest cylinder size used in anaesthesia is C, while the biggest is J. Air cylinders have white and black quartered shoulders and grey bodies. The pressure in a full nitrous oxide cylinder is 53 bar.

30. Lithium
- A. Potentiates non-depolarizing neuromuscular drugs
- B. Is an anion
- C. Toxicity is associated with tremor
- D. Chronic use can cause hyperthyroidism
- E. Causes the syndrome of inappropriate antidiuretic hormone release (SIADH)

31. Breathing 100% oxygen
- A. The PO_2 in arterial blood is 101.3 kPa
- B. Hypoxia due to shunt is dramatically improved
- C. The PO_2 of arterial blood in hyperbaric conditions of 2 atm will be double that at sea level
- D. The oxygen dissociation curve is shifted to the left
- E. The apparent functional capacity (AFC) of the lung is unaltered

30. TFTFF
A helpful tip! An anion is **a negative ion**. Lithium (Li^+) is a cation. It potentiates non-depolarizing muscle relaxants and can prolong the action of suxamethonium. Lithium has a low therapeutic index. Lithium mimics other cations, especially sodium, and makes the resting membrane potential more positive and more likely to depolarize. Therefore, tremor is a feature of toxicity. Other symptoms of mild toxicity include nausea, vomiting, abdominal pain, diarrhoea and sedation. Severe toxicity causes fits, hyperreflexia, coma and cardiac arrhythmias. Lithium inhibits thyroxine production so that hypothyroidism and goitre can occur. Lithium inhibits the action of antidiuretic hormone producing diabetes insipidus. Chronic toxicity can result in permanent renal and neurological damage.

31. FFFFF
The PO_2 of dry inspired air is 101.3 kPa. The PO_2 in arterial blood will be less than the PO_2 of inspired air due to the effect of water vapour. The SVP of water vapour at body temperature is 6.25 kPa. The arterial PO_2 will therefore be $100/100 \times (101.3 - 6.25)$ or 95.05 kPa (713 mmHg). Hypoxia due to a large shunt does not improve even when breathing 100% oxygen. At 2 atm the $PO_2 = 100/100 \times (202.6 - 6.25)$ or 196.35 kPa (compared to 95.05 kPa at 1 atm). The oxygen dissociation curve is unaffected by the inspired oxygen concentration. AFC stands for Arsenal Football Club. Watching Arsenal does indeed take the breath away and 100% oxygen is often required.

32. Regarding heat loss during anaesthesia
   A. The majority of heat loss is by convection
   B. Heat loss may be reduced by the use of heat and
      moisture exchangers
   C. Hypothermia results in hypercoaguability
   D. Hypothermia causes J waves on the ECG
   E. More oxygen is dissolved in the plasma of hypothermic
      than normothermic patients

33. Regarding intra-arterial blood pressure measurement
   A. The transducer system tubing should be compliant
   B. The natural frequency of the transducer system should
      be close to 20 Hz
   C. The cannula should be parallel sided and short
   D. An air bubble in the tubing increases the resonant
      frequency of the transducer system
   E. Under-damping will cause underestimation of the
      diastolic blood pressure

34. Concerning intraocular pressure
   A. Aqueous humour is formed by the ciliary body
   B. The normal intraocular pressure is 15 mmHg
   C. Suxamethonium increases intraocular pressure
   D. Aqueous humour drains into the posterior chamber of
      the eye via the canal of Schlemm
   E. Acetazolamide reduces intraocular pressure

32. FTFTT
Most heat is lost by radiation (60%). Heat loss by radiation is in the form of infrared waves from warm to cooler objects. About 10% of heat loss is due to warming and humidifying cool, dry inspired anaesthetic gases. Using heat and moisture exchangers reduces heat loss by this route. Hypothermia impairs blood clotting by reducing the activity of platelets and enzymes in the coagulation pathway. J waves are positive deflections at the end of the QRS complex and occur when the body temperature falls below 30°C. As the temperature of any liquid falls, more gas is dissolved in it. In normothermic patients 0.3 ml of oxygen is dissolved per 100 ml of plasma compared to 3.2 ml/100 ml when body temperature is 10°C.

33. FFTFT
Compliant tubing will absorb the pressure pulse being measured in the artery, damping the recording and causing underestimation of the true blood pressure. The transducer tubing should therefore be stiff. The natural frequency of a system is the frequency at which it resonates or rings. If the frequency of the pressure wave being measured is similar to the natural frequency of the system measuring it, the wave will be amplified. Therefore, to prevent amplification, the natural frequency of the transducer system should be much greater than the frequency of the waves being measured, which in the case of blood pressure is 20 Hz. Air bubbles in the tubing cause damping and reduce the resonant frequency of the transducer system towards 20 Hz. Under damping can result in overestimation of the systolic and underestimation of the diastolic blood pressure.

34. TTTFT
The ciliary body is found just behind the iris where the lens is attached to the eyeball. Aqueous humour flows into the anterior chamber and exits via the canal of Schlemm situated in the angle between the iris and cornea. The formation of aqueous humour is an active process and involves the enzyme carbonic anhydrase. Acetazolamide inhibits this enzyme and reduces intraocular pressure. It is therefore used in the treatment of glaucoma.

35. Regarding the biotransformation of drugs, the following are phase I reactions
  A. Oxidation
  B. Acetylation
  C. Hydrolysis
  D. Glucuronide conjugation
  E. Reduction

36. Concerning the components of breathing systems
  A. The external diameter of an adjustable pressure limiting valve is 22 mm
  B. The external diameter of endotracheal tube connectors is 13 mm
  C. The Mapleson C breathing system is a T-piece
  D. The Mapleson E breathing system always has a bag attachment
  E. The Cardiff swivel is a type of endotracheal tube connector

37. Regarding non-steroidal anti-inflammatory drugs (NSAIDs)
  A. NSAIDs are highly protein bound
  B. Ketorolac has a longer half-life than diclofenac
  C. Diclofenac is a selective cyclo-oxygenase-2 (COX-2) inhibitor
  D. The oral bioavailability of NSAIDs is greater than 60%
  E. Ketorolac and diclofenac, but not ibuprofen cause bronchospasm in asthmatic patients

38. Regarding features of a phase II neuromuscular block
  A. It usually follows a single dose of suxamethonium
  B. The train of four (TOF) ratio is > 0.7
  C. Tetanic fade is seen
  D. There is no post tetanic facilitation
  E. Phase II blockade is potentiated by anticholinesterases

35. TFTFT
Phase I reactions inactivate drugs. Phase II reactions, such as glucuronide conjugation and acetylation make water insoluble substances excretable.

36. TFFFF
The external diameter of endotracheal tube connectors is 15 mm. The Jackson Rees modification of the Mapleson E has a bag. This was originally used to detect respiration. The Cardiff swivel is the name given to a type of common gas outlet on anaesthetic machines.

37. TTFTF
NSAIDs are highly protein bound and can displace other protein bound drugs, e.g. sulphonylureas, warfarin and lithium. The half-lives of ketorolac and diclofenac are 300 min and 90 min, respectively. Diclofenac and paracetamol inhibit both COX-1 and COX-2 equally, while aspirin, indomethacin and ibuprofen are more specific inhibitors of COX-1. NSAIDs, other than diclofenac, undergo very limited first pass metabolism so the oral bioavailability is high. Diclofenac is metabolized to a large degree in the liver and has an oral bioavailability of only 60%. Ibuprofen also causes bronchospasm.

38. FFTFF
Phase II block sometimes follows repeated suxamethonium doses or infusion. The features of the block change from a depolarizing to a non-depolarizing block. The TOF ratio is < 0.3, there is post-tetanic facilitation and the block is antagonized by anticholinesterases.

39. Regarding electricity
   A. When a current of 1 ampere flows for 1 second in an electrical circuit, a charge of 1 coulomb will pass any point in that circuit
   B. The current flow through an electrical circuit is proportional to the resistance of the circuit
   C. The power generated by an electrical circuit is measured in joules
   D. Capacitors impede the passage of a direct current (DC) but allow the flow of an alternating current (AC)
   E. Mains voltage in the UK is 240 V

40. The following are physiological changes that occur in pregnancy
   A. Total blood volume increases by 45%
   B. Platelet concentration decreases by 20%
   C. Barrier pressure (lower oesophageal pressure (LOS) minus intragastric pressure) decreases
   D. Haematocrit decreases
   E. Plasma creatinine concentration increases

41. Regarding osmolarity
   A. The osmolarity of normal saline 0.9% solution is 150 mosmol/l
   B. Over 99% of the osmolarity of the plasma is due to plasma proteins
   C. The osmolarity of plasma is 200 mosmol/l
   D. The saturated vapour pressure (SVP) of a solvent increases the more solute is dissolved in it
   E. Osmolarity is measured using a hair hygrometer

39. TFFTT
You must know definitions of electrical terms. Ohm's law states that the current in an electrical circuit is proportional to the potential difference (V) and inversely proportional to the resistance (R), i.e. $I = V/R$. Power in an electrical circuit is measured in Watts.

40. TFTTF
Although there is an increased consumption of platelets in pregnancy, the platelet count usually remains unchanged although in some women it falls slightly. This is probably because there is increased platelet production. Due to a significant increase in intragastric pressure, the barrier pressure is reduced. Haematocrit falls due to the relatively greater increase in plasma volume as compared to the increase in red cell volume. Glomerular filtration rate increases in pregnancy resulting in a lower plasma creatinine.

41. FFFFF
In a solution the osmolarity is determined by the total molarity of the ions in that solution. In the case of normal saline 0.9%, this is 300 mosmol/l, i.e. Na^+ 150 mmol/l and Cl^- 150 mmol/l. Plasma proteins contribute about 1 mosmol/l to the total plasma osmolarity of approximately 300 mosmol/l. Over 99% of the plasma osmolarity comes from electrolytes such as sodium, chloride and bicarbonate. Raoult's law states that the fall in vapour pressure of a solvent is proportional to the molar concentration of the solute. This is because the more solute that is present in a solvent, the less surface area is available for evaporation, reducing the SVP. Osmolarity is measured using an osmometer. The hair hygrometer measures humidity.

42. Regarding opioid analgesics
  A. Opioid receptors are linked to G-proteins
  B. Pethidine prevents 5–HT re-uptake into nerve endings
  C. The OP_2 receptor is responsible for the dysphoria associated with opioids
  D. Diamorphine binds directly to OP_3 receptors to produce its effect
  E. The metabolites of pethidine are pharmacologically inactive

43. Regarding the ventricle of the heart
  A. The steeper the end diastolic pressure-volume curve, the lower the compliance of the ventricle during filling
  B. The Frank-Starling relationship is obtained if blood pressure is plotted against cardiac output
  C. The Frank-Starling curve is shifted down and to the right in a patient taking β-blockers
  D. The Frank-Starling curve is shifted down and to the right in a patient on nitrates
  E. The normal ejection fraction is 60–65%

42. TTTFF

Monoamine oxidase inhibitors (MAOIs) inhibit the breakdown of 5–HT while pethidine prevents its re-uptake into nerve endings. The result of giving pethidine to a patient who is either taking MAOIs or has stopped them within 2 weeks is blood pressure lability, agitation, rigidity and hyperpyrexia. Therefore, pethidine is contraindicated in this group of patients. The OP_2 receptor, formerly known as the κ receptor, causes dysphoria. The OP_1 receptor used to be called the δ receptor while the μ receptor is now called the OP_3 receptor. Both of these receptors cause, amongst other effects, euphoria. Diamorphine itself has no analgesic action, as it does not bind to opioid receptors. It is rapidly hydrolysed in the plasma and liver to produce mono-acetylmorphine which is then converted to morphine. Pethidine is converted to the active metabolite norpethidine in the liver. Norpethidine can cause hallucinations, fits and coma.

43. TFTFT

The pressure-volume curve for the ventricle describes the change in filling pressure per unit change in volume. The less compliant the ventricle the greater the required change in pressure to give the same change in volume, i.e. the steeper the curve. The Frank-Starling curve relates initial muscle fibre length to the tension developed by that muscle. A plot of any measure of initial fibre length, e.g. CVP, PAWP against any measure of cardiac output, e.g. stroke volume, blood pressure, will demonstrate the Frank-Starling relationship. Anything that decreases ventricular contractility will move the Frank-Starling curve down and to the right, while the opposite is true for factors that increase contractility.

44. Flow of fluid through a tube is more likely to be turbulent if:
  A. There is a sudden increase in the flow through the tube
  B. The viscosity of the fluid increases
  C. The density of the fluid increases
  D. Reynold's number is 200
  E. Heliox is breathed rather than air

45. Desflurane
  A. Desflurane has a lower oil/gas partition coefficient than halothane
  B. The desflurane vaporizer is heated to increase the volatility of desflurane
  C. Desflurane's low blood:gas partition coefficient makes it ideal to use for inhalational induction of anaesthesia
  D. 3–5% of desflurane is metabolized by the liver
  E. Desflurane does not sensitize the heart to circulating catecholamines

44. TFTFF

If Reynold's number is greater than 2000, then turbulent flow is likely. Reynold's number $= v\rho d/\eta$, where v is the linear velocity of the fluid, ρ is the density of the fluid, η is the viscosity of the fluid and d is the diameter of the tube. Thus, turbulence is more likely if viscosity of the fluid decreases. Heliox is less dense than air. Therefore, turbulent flow is less likely at a given flow rate breathing heliox rather than air.

45. TFFFT

The oil/gas partition coefficients of desflurane and halothane are 19 and 224, respectively. The SVP of desflurane at 20°C is high (88.5 kPa). It has a high volatility and a low boiling point compared to the other volatile agents (22.8°C). Therefore, in a standard vaporizer at room temperature the concentration of desflurane added to the fresh gas would be unpredictable as it would fluctuate with changes in ambient temperature, i.e. at 25°C desflurane would be boiling, while at 20°C it would not. By heating and pressurizing the vaporizer and injecting desflurane into the fresh gas under computer control the final concentration of desflurane in the breathing system is very accurate. The low blood/gas partition coefficient of desflurane means that end tidal and blood concentrations equilibrate rapidly so that induction of, and recovery from anaesthesia is quick. However, these properties are offset by the fact that desflurane is irritant to the airway and increases bronchial and salivary secretions which makes inhalational induction unpleasant for the patient and can result in laryngospasm. Although the blood/gas partition coefficient of sevoflurane is slightly higher (0.69), it is far less irritant and is ideal for inhalational induction, particularly in children. Desflurane is 0.02% metabolized.

46. The following impair hypoxic pulmonary vasoconstriction
A. Acidosis
B. Cyclo-oxygenase inhibitors
C. Volatile anaesthetic agents
D. Bronchodilators
E. Nitrates

47. Regarding exponential functions
A. After three half-lives 6.25% of the initial amount of a substance will remain
B. The time constant is shorter than the half-life
C. After one time constant 37% of the initial amount of a substance will remain
D. The nitrogen washout curve is exponential
E. All exponential processes are negative

48. Etomidate
A. Etomidate is insoluble in water but is soluble in propylene glycol
B. Etomidate inhibits the enzyme 11,β-hydroxylase
C. Etomidate is contraindicated in patients with porphyria
D. In the plasma etomidate is 5–10% protein bound
E. Etomidate has an elimination half-life of 75 min

49. The following regarding pressure are true
A. The pressure inside a full entonox cylinder is 137 bar
B. The critical pressure of oxygen is 50 bar
C. Suction equipment should generate a negative pressure of at least 2.5 bar
D. The pressure of piped medical air is 4 bar
E. Normal atmospheric pressure at sea level is 750 mmHg

46. FFTTT
Acidosis and cyclo-oxygenase inhibitors potentiate hypoxic pulmonary vasoconstriction. Other drugs that impair hypoxic pulmonary vasoconstriction include nitroprusside and calcium channel blockers.

47. FFTTF
Exponential processes can be positive or negative depending on whether the substance concerned is increasing or decreasing in amount. The nitrogen washout curve is a negative exponential process as the amount of nitrogen in the lungs falls exponentially when 100% oxygen is breathed. After three half-lives, 12.5% of a substance will remain, i.e. half of a half of a half or one-eighth (100 → 50 → 25 → 12.5). The time constant is the time at which the process would have been completed had the initial rate of change continued. It is longer than a half-life.

48. FTTFT
Etomidate is soluble but unstable in water so that it is dissolved in a mixture of water and propylene glycol. 11,β-hydroxylase is required for steroid synthesis. The inhibition of steroid synthesis by etomidate is only clinically relevant during infusions, e.g. ITU. It is no longer licensed to be given by this route. You should know the list of unsafe drugs in porphyria and will find an excellent question in this book that lists many of them. Etomidate is 76% protein bound.

49. TTFTF
The critical pressure is the pressure required to liquefy a vapour at its critical temperature. The British standard for medical vacuum systems requires that they should generate a negative pressure of at least 533 mbar and a flow rate of 40 l/min. The pressure in all pipeline gases for the anaesthetic machine is 4 bar. However medical air used to drive instruments such as drills is at 7 bar. The normal atmospheric pressure is 760 mmHg or 101.33 kPa.

50. Regarding the transfusion of blood
    A. Anti-A is an IgM antibody
    B. 3% of the UK population are blood group AB
    C. Anti-Rhesus D (RhD) antibodies formed in a RhD-negative recipient of RhD-positive blood are IgG antibodies
    D. Patients with blood group AB can safely receive group A blood
    E. Dextran infusions interfere with blood cross-matching

51. Dantrolene
    A. Is a white powder
    B. Has a low water solubility
    C. Prevents calcium from binding to troponin C
    D. The initial dose of dantrolene in a patient with malignant hyperpyrexia is 1 mg/kg
    E. A solution of dantrolene has a shelf life of 24 h

52. Regarding the neuromuscular junction
    A. The acetylcholine receptor consists of five subunits
    B. Acetylcholine is formed from pyruvate
    C. Acetylcholine binds to the α subunit of the acetylcholine receptor
    D. The resting membrane potential of skeletal muscle is −60 mV
    E. Calcium reduces the release of acetylcholine from motor neurones

50. TTTTT
Antibodies to ABO antigens are IgM. Anti-RhD antibodies are IgG and can therefore cross the placenta to cause haemolytic disease of the newborn. 47% of the UK population are blood group O, 42% are group A and 8% are group B. The percentages are different in other populations. People who are blood group AB have no naturally occurring Anti-A or Anti-B antibodies and can therefore receive blood of any ABO group.

51. FTFTF
Dantrolene sodium is an orange powder that is presented in bottles, which contain 20 mg of dantrolene, 3 g of mannitol and some sodium hydroxide. 60 ml of water is added to prepare the intravenous solution, which then has a shelf life of only 6 h. As dantrolene is very poorly soluble in water, reconstituting it can take a long time. Dantrolene prevents calcium release from the sarcoplasmic reticulum.

52. TTTFF
The acetylcholine receptor is made of five polypeptide subunits arranged like a cylinder with a central channel. When acetylcholine binds to the α subunit the cylinder becomes more permeable to sodium ions and an action potential is set up in the muscle. Acetylcholine is formed from Acetyl-Co A and choline. Acetyl-Co A is formed from pyruvate. The resting membrane potential in cardiac pacemaker cells is –60 mV. It is –90 mV in skeletal muscle cells. Calcium increases the release of acetylcholine from motor neurones.

53. Regarding pulse oximetry
A. A pulse oximeter contains a single light emitting diode (LED)
B. The LED emits light at a wavelength of 805 nm
C. The isobestic wavelength of oxy- and deoxyhaemoglobin is 940 nm
D. The LED emits dichromatic light
E. The pulse oximeter is most accurate over the saturation range of 50–100%

54. The alkalinization of urine increases the excretion of the following
A. Acidic drugs
B. Aspirin
C. Ephedrine
D. Amphetamine
E. Phenobarbitone

55. Regarding the movement of fluid in and out of capillaries
A. The hydrostatic pressure at the arterial end of a systemic capillary is 45 mmHg
B. The colloid osmotic pressure in a systemic capillary is 10 mmHg
C. The interstitial colloid osmotic pressure at the venous end of a capillary is 3 times that at the arterial end
D. Vasoconstriction reduces the rate of filtration at the arterial end of the capillary
E. Capillaries contain 35% of the circulating blood volume

53. FFFFF

A pulse oximeter consists of two LEDs which each emit monochromatic light, one at a wavelength of 660 nm (red) and the other at 940 nm (infrared). At these wavelengths the absorbance of light by oxy- and deoxyhaemoglobin are markedly different. The isobestic points for oxy- and deoxyhaemoglobin, i.e. where the absorbance properties are the same, are 590 nm and 805 nm. It is important to know these four wavelengths as they always crop up in MCQs. Oximeters are calibrated from information obtained from previous human studies. As it is unethical to desaturate a volunteer to 50%, calibration at these low oxygen saturations is extrapolated. Pulse oximeters are most accurate over a range of 80–100%.

54. TTFFT

For acidic drugs the Henderson-Hasselbach equation states that: $pH = pKa + \log_{10}$ [ionized drug]/[unionized drug]. In the proximal and distal tubules, unionized forms of weak acids and bases are reabsorbed. Therefore, manipulation of the urinary pH can alter the amount of drug that is absorbed and excreted. Changing the pH of urine from 6.4 to 8 increases the excretion of acidic drugs, e.g. aspirin ($pKa = 3.5$) and phenobarbitone ($pKa = 7.2$). Amphetamine is a basic drug (i.e. $pH = pKa + \log_{10}$ [unionized]/[ionized]) and is excreted to a greater degree in an acidic urine, although this has little clinical effect.

55. FFFTF

The hydrostatic pressures at the arterial and venous ends of capillaries are 33 mmHg and 15 mmHg, respectively. The interstitial hydrostatic pressure is about 1 mmHg, although it varies from tissue to tissue. The colloid osmotic pressure in the capillary is 25 mmHg, while in the interstitium it is zero. Starling's forces favouring inward or outward movements of fluid depend on the magnitude of these pressures. Vasoconstriction reduces the hydrostatic pressure at the arterial end of the capillary, which in turn reduces the amount of fluid forced into the interstitium. Capillaries contain 6% of the circulating blood volume.

56. The following measure gas flow rate
   A. Rotameter
   B. Vitalograph
   C. Pneumotachograph
   D. Wright respirometer
   E. Haldane apparatus

57. Regarding antiemetics
   A. Cyclizine causes bronchoconstriction
   B. Prochlorperazine causes bradycardia
   C. Droperidol is a phenothiazine
   D. Ondansetron increases prolactin secretion
   E. Metoclopramide is 90% protein bound

58. Regarding glomerular filtration rate (GFR)
   A. The normal GFR is 125 ml/min
   B. *Para*-aminohippuric (PAH) acid is used to measure GFR
   C. The hydrostatic pressure in the glomerular capillary falls along its length
   D. The hydrostatic pressure at the afferent arteriolar end of the glomerular capillary is 45 mmHg
   E. Creatinine clearance underestimates GFR

59. The following are base SI units
   A. Coulomb
   B. Joule
   C. Newton
   D. Ohm
   E. Mole

56. TTTFF
The pneumotachograph measures the fall in pressure as a gas flows through it and relates this using Poiseuille's (a surgeon!!) law to flow rate. The Wright respirometer uses a spinning vane to measure expired volume. Flow can only be deduced from it over a period of time. The Haldane apparatus is used to measure the components in a mixture of gases.

57. FFFFF
Cyclizine has no effect on the respiratory system. Prochlorperazine is a phenothiazine and therefore has some α-blocking properties. It can cause hypotension with a compensatory tachycardia. Droperidol is a butyrophenone and blocks D_2 receptors in the chemoreceptor trigger zone. Ondansetron has no effect on prolactin secretion. Metoclopramide is 18% protein bound while droperidol is 90% bound to protein.

58. TFFTF
Inulin is used to measure GFR while PAH determines renal plasma flow. Due to the efferent arteriole which acts as a second resistance vessel, the hydrostatic pressure in the glomerular capillary remains at 45 mmHg throughout its entire length. Like inulin, creatinine is easily filtered in the glomerulus. However, unlike inulin, creatinine is secreted by the renal tubule so that creatinine clearance tends to be higher than inulin clearance.

59. FFFFT
There are seven base SI units. They are: metre (length), kilogram (mass), second (time), candela (light), ampere (electrical current), kelvin (temperature) and mole (quantity). The definitions of the other derived units in this question appear elsewhere in this book.

60. Tramadol
   A. The oral dose of tramadol is 50–100 mg given 4–6 hourly
   B. Tramadol is a μ receptor agonist
   C. Tramadol is contraindicated in patients taking monoamine oxidase inhibitors (MAOIs)
   D. The metabolites of tramadol are inactive
   E. Tramadol has a direct effect on GABA and NMDA receptors

61. Regarding the normal Valsalva manoeuvre
   A. Initially the blood pressure falls
   B. Heart rate tends to rise
   C. The first change in cardiac output is a rise
   D. Immediately after the glottis is opened blood pressure falls
   E. The Valsalva manoeuvre may be abnormal in diabetics

62. Regarding intravenous anaesthetic drugs
   A. 30% of a dose of thiopentone remains in the body after 24 h
   B. The elimination half-life ($T_{1/2}\beta$) of thiopentone is 5–10 h
   C. Propofol is 1,6–di-isopropyl phenol
   D. Diazepam is water soluble
   E. The pH in an ampoule of midazolam is 3

63. Regarding closed-circuit breathing systems
   A. Dangerously high concentrations of anaesthetic vapours can be given to the patient
   B. The Waters' canister is a closed-circuit breathing system
   C. Barium lime is more efficient than soda lime in absorbing carbon dioxide
   D. Clayton yellow changes from yellow to white as soda lime is exhausted
   E. 100 g of soda lime can absorb 26 l of carbon dioxide

60. TTTFF

Tramadol is a weak agonist at all opioid receptors but is most selective for the µ receptor. Tramadol blocks the re-uptake of noradrenaline and 5–HT so its use in patients taking, or having stopped MAOIs within 2 weeks, is contraindicated. A metabolite of tramadol, O-desmethyltramadol, has a greater analgesic potency than tramadol and a half-life of 9 h.

61. FTTTT

Following a forced expiration against a closed glottis blood pressure increases as the rise in intrathoracic pressure is transmitted to the aorta. The first change in cardiac output is a transient rise as blood is forced from the pulmonary veins into the left atrium. After the initial increase in blood pressure, it begins to fall as venous return and cardiac output fall. There is a reflex tachycardia. Any cause of autonomic neuropathy, e.g. diabetes, can cause an abnormal cardiovascular response to the Valsalva manoeuvre.

62. TTFFT

Propofol is 2,6–di-isopropyl phenol. Diazepam is dissolved either in propylene glycol or a soya bean lipid emulsion, as it is insoluble in water.

63. TFFFT

Anaesthetic vapour can accumulate in circle systems particularly with the vaporizor in circle if the fresh gas flow is very low. The less soluble the vapour is in the blood, the less will be taken up by the patient and the higher the concentration in the breathing system. The Waters' canister is a cylindrical drum that contains soda lime. It is classified as a Mapleson C breathing system and is therefore not a closed circuit. Barium lime is 15% less efficient than soda lime. As carbon dioxide is absorbed the pH of soda lime decreases, which turns Clayton yellow from a deep pink colour when the soda lime is fresh to off-white. Ethyl violet, another indicator turns from colourless to violet when the soda lime is exhausted.

64. Regarding nausea and vomiting
- A. The chemoreceptor trigger zone (CTZ) lies within the blood-brain barrier
- B. The CTZ contains opioid (μ) receptors
- C. The vomiting centre responds to vagal afferents from the gastrointestinal tract
- D. Ondansetron acts only on the CTZ
- E. $5-HT_2$ receptors are found in the CTZ

65. Regarding anaesthetic machines
- A. Pressure reducing valves provide a constant gas pressure of about 4 bar
- B. The oxygen flush should deliver oxygen at a flow rate of at least 20 l/min
- C. The Bosun whistle is a suitable oxygen failure warning device
- D. The pressure relief valve at the end of the back bar protects the patient from barotrauma
- E. The Bodok seal prevents leakage of anaesthetic vapour from the attachment of the vaporizer to the back bar

66. Regarding the immune response
- A. Cytokines are phospholipids
- B. Lymphocytes are the first white cells to migrate to sites of injury
- C. Tumour necrosis factor (TNF) is produced by endothelial cells in response to injury
- D. Type I hypersensitivity reactions are mediated by IgG
- E. Type IV hypersensitivity is seen in patients who are allergic to penicillin and are given penicillin

64. FTTFF

The CTZ lies outside the blood-brain barrier in the area postrema in the fourth ventricle. The CTZ has opioid (μ), serotonergic (5-HT$_3$), adrenergic (α_1 and α_2) and dopaminergic (D$_2$) receptors. The vomiting centre is located in the dorsolateral reticular formation, inside the blood-brain barrier, and has 5-HT$_3$, D$_2$ and muscarinic (M$_3$) receptors. Therefore, opioids act only on the CTZ, while ondansetron, a 5-HT$_3$ antagonist, acts on both. The vomiting centre, but not the CTZ, receives vagal afferents.

65. TFFFF

The oxygen flush should provide oxygen at a flow rate of at least 35 l/min. The Bosun whistle can be switched off and requires a battery that can run out. These features make it unsuitable. The downstream pressure relief valve on the back bar blows off at 38–40 kPa and protects the rotameters from over pressure. The Bodok seal is a washer between the cylinder and yoke and prevents leakage of gas.

66. FFFFF

Cytokines are peptides or glycopeptides. One type of cytokine is TNF, which is produced by macrophages and lymphocytes in response to bacterial infection. It increases vascular permeability and adhesiveness and increases the bacteriocidal effects of macrophages. Neutrophils are the first cells to adhere to endothelial cells and migrate into the interstium at the site of injury. Type I hypersensitivity reactions, which are mediated by IgE, occur in previously sensitized individuals and can cause anaphylactic shock. Type IV hypersensitivity reactions are cell-mediated and occur at least 12 h after exposure to the antigen, e.g. the response to tuberculin injection.

67. Regarding the Magill breathing system
   A. During spontaneous ventilation, exhaled alveolar gas exits through the valve
   B. The Magill breathing system is classified as a Mapleson D
   C. To prevent rebreathing in a spontaneously breathing patient the fresh gas flow rate should be equal to or greater than the minute ventilation
   D. The Humphrey system is a co-axial Magill circuit
   E. The expiratory valve is at the patient end

68. Clonidine
   A. Increases blood pressure
   B. Is a bronchodilator
   C. Reduces the MAC of volatile anaesthetic drugs
   D. Decreases blood pressure
   E. Is an α_2 antagonist

69. Regarding the carriage of carbon dioxide in the blood
   A. Carbonic anhydrase is found in the red blood cell and the plasma
   B. Carbon dioxide is mostly transported as carbamino compounds in the blood
   C. Oxyhaemoglobin is more able to carry carbon dioxide than deoxyhaemoglobin
   D. Carbon dioxide is less soluble in the blood than oxygen
   E. When carbonic acid dissociates into bicarbonate and hydrogen ions, chloride ions diffuse out of the red blood cell with hydrogen to maintain electrical neutrality

67. TFFFT

The Magill attachment is a Mapleson A. As alveolar gas passes out through the expiratory valve during expiration and dead space gas passes down the tubing, the following inspired breath does not contain carbon dioxide. This makes the Magill system efficient when breathing spontaneously. The fresh gas flow rate needs to be at least equal to the alveolar ventilation, i.e. 70 ml/kg/min to prevent rebreathing of carbon dioxide. As the valve is closed during positive pressure ventilation, carbon dioxide will accumulate as it cannot escape. The Magill is inefficient therefore in the ventilated patient. The Lack system is a co-axial Magill. The expiratory valve and the bag are at the machine end in a Humphrey ADE system, which also has a lever within the valve block that converts it into either a Mapleson A, D or E type of circuit.

68. TFTTF

Clonidine is an α_2 agonist and reduces blood pressure by a central action preventing noradrenaline release. It has a transient α_1 agonist effect which increases blood pressure. Clonidine has no effect on the lungs.

69. FFFFF

Carbon dioxide is mainly transported in the blood as bicarbonate ions. It is also carried as carbamino compounds bound to blood proteins, and dissolved in plasma. It is 20 times more soluble than oxygen. Carbonic anhydrase is only present in red blood cells and catalyses the formation of carbonic acid from carbon dioxide and water. Carbonic acid quickly dissociates into hydrogen and bicarbonate ions. The cell membrane is relatively impermeable to cations so that hydrogen ions do not readily diffuse out into the plasma. Bicarbonate however diffuses readily. Chloride ions replace bicarbonate ions in the red blood cell to maintain electrical neutrality. This is the chloride shift. The hydrogen ions formed by the dissociation of carbonic acid combine with reduced haemoglobin as it is a better proton acceptor than oxyhaemoglobin. The presence of reduced haemoglobin therefore promotes the carriage of carbon dioxide. This is known as the Haldane effect.

70. Regarding the scavenging of anaesthetic gases
  A. Scavenging tubing has 30 mm connections
  B. An assisted passive disposal system uses the air conditioning's extractor ducts
  C. Active disposal systems require high pressure, high volume extractor fans
  D. Hospital suction is suitable for use in active disposal systems
  E. In passive systems, resistance to flow should be less than 10 cmH$_2$O

71. Neostigmine
  A. Causes bronchospasm
  B. Reduces salivary secretions
  C. 90% of a dose of neostigmine is hydrolysed by the liver
  D. Is a quaternary amine
  E. Reduces anatomical dead space

72. The following can be compressed into liquids at room temperature
  A. Xenon
  B. Air
  C. Entonox
  D. Heliox
  E. Nitrogen

73. Aldosterone
  A. Spironolactone is an aldosterone antagonist
  B. Increases tubular secretion of sodium
  C. Is produced in the adrenal cortex
  D. Increases renal blood flow
  E. Promotes hydrogen loss in the kidney

70. TTFFF
30 mm connectors prevent accidental connection to other parts of the breathing circuit. Active disposal systems require low pressure, high volume extractor fans capable of removing 75 l/min with a peak flow of 130 l/min. Hospital suction apparatus provides a minimal flow rate of about 40 l/min and is thus inadequate for use in an active scavenging system. In passive systems the resistance to flow should be no more than 0.5 cmH₂O at a flow of 30 l/min.

71. TFFTT
Neostigmine increases acetylcholine concentrations at nerve endings. It is therefore parasympathomimetic, increasing salivary secretions, causing bronchoconstriction and reducing dead space. It is mainly hydrolysed by acetylcholine esterase and plasma cholinesterase and 60% appears in the urine. A small percentage is metabolized by the liver and excreted in the bile.

72. FFFFF
Gases can not be compressed into a liquid whatever the pressure applied, whereas vapours can. If the critical temperature (CT) of a substance is less than the surrounding temperature then it is a gas and cannot be compressed into a liquid. The CTs of vapours on the other hand are greater than the ambient temperature. Therefore, at room temperature, nitrous oxide (CT, 34°C) and carbon dioxide (CT, 31°C) are vapours and can be compressed into liquids.

73. TFTFT
Aldosterone is released in response to a fall in plasma volume via the renin-angiotensin system, specifically in response to angiotensin II. It causes sodium reabsorption and hydrogen and potassium loss in the distal nephron. Aldosterone does not directly affect renal blood flow.

74. **The following statements regarding heat are true**
    A. The specific heat capacity is the heat energy required to raise the temperature of a unit mass of a substance by 1 kelvin
    B. The unit of specific heat capacity is J/K
    C. The copper heat sink in a vaporizer has a low specific heat capacity
    D. The latent heat capacity of a substance is the amount of heat energy required to change its state without a change in temperature
    E. The specific heat capacity of gases is less than that of liquids

75. **Adenosine**
    A. Intravenous adenosine should be administered as a slow bolus injection
    B. Adenosine is contraindicated in patients who are taking β-blockers
    C. Adenosine is a bronchodilator
    D. Adenosine causes nausea
    E. Adenosine slows A-V nodal conduction

76. **Regarding the liver**
    A. Conjugation of drugs in the liver is an example of phase I metabolism
    B. Vitamin K is required for the synthesis of factor IX
    C. Plasma albumin is a useful marker of acute liver injury
    D. 50% of patients who receive halothane show a rise in glutathione s-transferase
    E. The liver is the primary site for glycogen synthesis

77. **Regarding cerebral blood flow**
    A. The effect of arterial PaO_2 on cerebral blood flow is more marked than $PaCO_2$
    B. Cerebral blood flow is normally 55 ml/100 g/min
    C. White matter receives a higher proportion of cerebral blood flow than grey matter
    D. Jugular venous blood is 75% saturated with oxygen
    E. Cerebral blood flow decreases during convulsions

74. TFFTT
The unit of heat capacity is J/K. The unit of specific heat capacity is J/kg/K. Copper has a high specific heat capacity so that it can transfer heat energy into vaporizer chambers as heat is lost by evaporation without changing temperature. By maintaining the temperature, the vapour pressure of the volatile agent inside the vaporizer is kept constant.

75. FFFFT
As adenosine has a very short half-life (8–10 s), it must be administered quickly. It can be given safely in patients taking β-blockers. Stimulation of the A_1 adenosine receptor slows A-V nodal conduction and causes bronchoconstriction. Adenosine does not cause nausea.

76. FTFTT
Phase I metabolic reactions of drugs include oxidation, hydrolysis, hydration and reduction. Conjugation, e.g. with glucuronide, is a phase II reaction. Vitamin K is required for the synthesis of factors II, VII, IX and X. Clotting abnormality occurs early in liver impairment. This is because bile salts are required for the absorption of vitamin K from the bowel and some clotting factors have a very short half-life, e.g. factor VII has a half-life of 4 h. Albumin has a half-life of 20 days and is therefore not a good marker of acute liver injury. Although halothane is no longer widely used in the UK, its effect on the liver is important to understand.

77. FTFFF
Arterial $PaCO_2$ has a far greater effect on cerebral blood flow than arterial PaO_2. Grey matter has a blood flow of 70 ml/100 g/min compared to only 30 ml/100g/min for white matter. Jugular venous blood is only 65% saturated with oxygen as the brain has a high oxygen consumption of 3.5 ml/100 g/min. Cerebral perfusion increases greatly during fits.

78. The following should be avoided in patients with porphyria
   A. Ketamine
   B. Thiopentone
   C. Pancuronium
   D. Droperidol
   E. Lidocaine

79. The following sterilize anaesthetic equipment
   A. Pasteurization for 20 min at 70°C
   B. 0.1–0.5% chlorhexidine
   C. Autoclave
   D. 70% alcohol
   E. 2% gluteraldehyde

80. Daily nutritional requirements for a resting adult are
   A. Proteins 1 g/kg
   B. Carbohydrates 0.5 g/kg
   C. Fat 0.5 g/kg
   D. Sodium 1–2 mmol/kg
   E. Potassium 1 mmol/kg

78. FTTFF
Porphyrias are a group of conditions in which one or more of the enzymes responsible for the synthesis of haem is defective causing a build up of precursors in the haem pathway. Many of the drugs that precipitate porphyria are inducers of hepatic cytochrome P–450, which is the main consumer of haem in the liver. Induction of cytochrome P–450 therefore depletes the haem pool, with loss of negative feedback on aminolaevulinate (ALA) synthetase, the first enzyme in the synthesis of haem from succinyl CoA and glycine. This increases the rate of haem production and the build up of haem precursors in patients with porphyria. The list of unsafe drugs is long and varied. It is difficult to remember them all but unfortunately easy to ask MCQs about. Pentazocine, chlordiazepoxide, etomidate, pancuronium, steroids, griseofulvin, alcohol, thiopentone, the contraceptive pill, prochlorperazine, chloramphenicol, sulphonamides, alpha-methyldopa, flunitrazepam, phenytoin and chlorpropamide are unsafe in porphyria.

79. FFTFF
A, B, D and E disinfect, i.e. they kill most organisms but not spores. Sterilization kills all organisms and spores. Gamma-irradiation, autoclave and ethylene oxide sterilize.

80. TFFTT
The daily requirements for proteins, carbohydrates and fat are 1, 2 and 2 g/kg, respectively.

81. Regarding the measurement of carbon dioxide (CO_2)
   A. The Severinghaus CO_2 electrode measures the change in pH of a bicarbonate solution
   B. pH changes linearly with the pCO_2
   C. The CO_2 electrode must be kept at a constant temperature
   D. CO_2 absorbs infrared light at a wavelength of 4.28 μm
   E. The absorption band of halothane overlaps that of CO_2

82. Naloxone
   A. Naloxone is a derivative of naltrexone
   B. Naloxone reverses the effect of buprenorphine
   C. The half-life of naloxone is 1–2 h
   D. Pulmonary oedema can occur after its use
   E. Naloxone has no therapeutic activity

83. The following are secondary messengers in cells
   A. ATP
   B. Cyclic AMP
   C. Calcium
   D. Cyclic GMP
   E. Diacylglycerol (DAG)

81. TFTTF

The CO_2 electrode consists of pH-sensitive glass dipped into a solution of bicarbonate. The pH of the bicarbonate solution varies depending on the amount of CO_2 that diffuses into it from the blood sample through a semi-permeable membrane. The pH inside the pH sensitive glass tube is kept constant. The potential difference between the bicarbonate solution and the inside of the pH sensitive glass is measured with two electrodes. As pH changes linearly with the log of the pCO_2, the CO_2 electrode can be calibrated to measure CO_2. Nitrous oxide absorbs light at a wavelength of 4.4 μm, which overlaps the absorption spectrum of CO_2. Halothane absorbs light in the ultraviolet range, i.e. light with a wavelength of 200 nm.

82. FFTTT

Naloxone is the *N*-allyl derivative of oxymorphone. Naltrexone is derived from naloxone and has similar effects but with a longer half-life (24 h). Naloxone does not reverse the effects of buprenorphine. Pulmonary oedema, tachycardia and cardiac arrest can occur following reversal of large doses of opioids and are thought to be due to the sudden release of catecholamines. Naloxone is a competitive agonist at opioid receptors. It has no clinical effect at this receptor. It simply reverses the effect of opioids. It therefore has a high affinity but an efficacy of 0.

83. FTTTT

Secondary messengers are released following receptor stimulation. They exert their effect by activating intracellular enzymes, in particular protein kinases. Calcium binds to intracellular proteins such as troponin and calmodulin. DAG is formed from phosphatidyl inositol diphosphate and activates protein kinase C. Phosphatidyl inositol diphosphate is the precursor for another secondary messenger, inositol triphosphate, which is involved in the release of calcium from the endoplasmic reticulum. Cyclic AMP, formed from ATP, influences the synthesis of DNA, RNA and proteins, and the breakdown of lipid and glycogen.

84. **Concerning vaporizers**
    A. The saturated vapour pressure of halothane at 20°C is 32 kPa at an atmospheric pressure of 100 kPa
    B. The EMO vaporizer uses a bimetallic strip for temperature compensation
    C. The saturated vapour pressure of halothane is 64 kPa at an atmospheric pressure of 200 kPa
    D. Plenum vaporizers have a high resistance to gas flow
    E. The Oxford Miniature Vaporizer (OMV) is used with ether

85. **Metoclopramide**
    A. Is a dopamine receptor antagonist
    B. Is anticholinergic
    C. Is a partial 5–HT_4 receptor agonist
    D. Has no effect on histamine (H_1) receptors
    E. Is chemically related to procaine

86. **With respect to Hartmann's solution**
    A. The pH is 6
    B. Does not contain calcium
    C. The sodium content is 131 mmol/l
    D. The chloride content is 131 mmol/l
    E. The lactate content is 39 mmol/l

87. **Sulphonylureas**
    A. Metformin is a sulphonylurea
    B. Sulphonylureas stimulate insulin secretion from the pancreas
    C. Chlorpropamide has a longer half-life than tolbutamide
    D. Aspirin augments the action of sulphonylureas
    E. Sulphonylureas reduce hepatic gluconeogenesis

84. TFFTF
Saturated vapour pressure is unaffected by the ambient pressure. Therefore, the SVP of halothane at an atmospheric pressure of 200 kPa is 32 kPa. For temperature compensation the EMO has a small bellows filled with ether which expands or contracts depending on the surrounding temperature thus opening or closing a valve. Gas is forced into plenum vaporizers under pressure and passes through a series of wicks from which anaesthetic vapour evaporates. The wicks increase the resistance to flow. The OMV is used with halothane, trilene or enflurane.

85. TFTFT
Metoclopramide is a D_2 receptor antagonist in the chemoreceptor trigger zone. It also has a weak affinity for the H_1 receptor and in high doses is a $5\text{–}HT_3$ receptor antagonist. It has no effect on muscarinic receptors. Metoclopramide is a partial $5\text{–}HT_4$ receptor agonist and its prokinetic actions may be mediated through these receptors in the gut wall.

86. TFTFF
You must know the content of all the intravenous fluids you give to patients. Read the bags during lists. The concentrations of ions in Hartmann's solution are Na^+ 131 mmol/l, K^+ 5 mmol/l, Ca^{2+} 2 mmol/l, lactate 29 mmol/l and Cl^- 111 mmol/l.

87. FTTTF
Metformin is a biguanide. Sulphonylureas stimulate insulin secretion from the α cells of the pancreas. Chlorpropamide (half-life 35 h), tolbutamide (half-life 5 h), glibenclamide and glicazide are examples of sulphonylureas. Aspirin, and other highly protein-bound drugs, increase the action of sulphonylureas by displacing them from albumin binding sites. The mode of action of biguanides is to reduce hepatic gluconeogenesis and increase glucose uptake in the periphery.

88. Magnesium
   A. The normal plasma concentration is 4 mmol/l
   B. Hypomagnesaemia causes delayed A-V conduction
   C. Hypomagnesaemia causes U waves on the ECG
   D. Hypomagnesaemia causes widening of the QRS complex of the ECG
   E. Magnesium relaxes bronchial smooth muscle

89. Concerning the normal electroencephalogram (EEG)
   A. δ waves are seen during sleep
   B. α waves have higher amplitudes than δ waves
   C. β waves are seen in patients with severe organic brain disease
   D. χ waves have a lower frequency than β waves
   E. α waves occur most intensely in the occipital region of the brain

90. Amiodarone
   A. Is a class III antiarrhythmic drug
   B. The initial intravenous dose is 50 μg/kg
   C. Has a half-life of 4 days
   D. Can cause irreversible corneal microdeposits
   E. Causes a rise in tri-iodothyronine levels

88. FFTFT
The normal plasma magnesium is 1.1 mmol/l.
Hypomagnesaemia is associated with increased myocardial
excitability and tachyarrhythmias, e.g. atrial fibrillation.
ECG changes include U waves, and peaked T waves.
Hypermagnesaemia causes delayed A-V conduction, a
prolonged PR interval and wide QRS complex. Magnesium
is useful in the treatment of asthma.

89. TFFTT
According to frequency, highest first, the order of the brain
waves is as follows: β (>14 Hz), α (8–13 Hz), χ (4–7 Hz) and
δ (<4 Hz). As the frequencies fall, the amplitudes rise. α
waves are seen in the awake and relaxed subject. β waves are
seen in people performing mental tasks. χ waves are seen in
children and in some adults under emotional stress. They
are also present in patients with brain disorders. δ waves are
seen during deep sleep and in patients with serious organic
brain disease.

90. TFFFT
Amiodarone acts by prolonging the cardiac action
potential and refractory period. The intravenous dose of
amiodarone is 5 mg/kg over 20–120 min followed by up to
15 mg/kg/24 h. The half-life is 4 weeks. The corneal
microdeposits are reversible and rarely affect vision.
Amiodarone is de-iodinated in the body and can cause a
rise in tri-iodothyronine levels by blocking the conversion of
thyroxine.

91. Regarding Arsenal Football Club
   A. Arsenal station on the Piccadilly line of the London tube network was formerly known as Gillespie Road
   B. Arsenal beat Manchester United in the 1979 FA Cup final
   C. The sun always shines on Highbury
   D. Arsenal have been in the top division of English football longer than any other team
   E. Arsenal is life, the rest is just detail

91. TTTTT

London Transport changed the name of Gillespie Road tube station to Arsenal, following the fantastic success of the team in the 1930s and a request from the inspirational manager Herbert Chapman. Incidentally a bust of Herbert Chapman can be seen in the famed marble halls of the East Stand at Highbury, a 'must see' for any visitor to London. Highbury is the home of football and by definition the sun always shines there. Arsenal crushed and humiliated Manchester United in the FA Cup final in 1979 winning the game comfortably 3–2. Arsenal has been in the top flight of English football since 1919, far far longer than any other team. In fact Henry Norris, the then manager engineered Arsenal's promotion to Division 1 at the expense of Tottenham despite being 5th in Division 2! (Gotta Laugh). Stem E has been copied straight out of the Final FRCA multiple choice questions book by Brunner, Robinson and Williams published by Butterworth Heinemann. We apologize, therefore, for asking a final FRCA standard question in this primary book, however, ARSENAL IS LIFE, THE REST IS JUST DETAIL.

3   The Vivas

There is no doubt that sitting face-to-face with your examiners across a table strewn with photographs, paper and pencils is one of the most, if not the most, stressful parts of the whole examination and, indeed, a candidate's whole life! For a start, it can often be somewhat intimidating to see the famous 'names' you have read or heard about so close up. To make matters worse, you are acutely aware of your own body exuding fear and tension, whilst the examiners themselves appear cool and relaxed. Once again, examiners are normal people with normal lives, so you must try to forget the idea that they hold your future career in the palms of their hands and have the ability to screw it into a ball and toss it over their shoulder without any apparent concern, leaving you helpless and wretched with nothing to look forward to except further pain and misery.

THE NATURE OF THE VIVAS

The vivas are held over several days and there is no significance to which day is selected for any particular candidate. There are two vivas, held on the same day, with the added pleasure of the OSCE to fit in as well. Each cohort of candidates receives the same questions and great pains are taken to ensure that there is no passing on of tips to the next cohort (the subjects are changed whenever one cohort leaves the examination halls and might 'contaminate' a 'virgin' cohort). The viva subjects are altered each day, and the examiners only see each day's subjects on the very morning and could be faced with asking questions on subjects about which they have only moderate knowledge. The examiners are provided with a list of questions to ask (in any order) and some structured related information to be used as guidance. Each candidate is supposed to answer all the questions, so waffling on for ages is generally a bad thing; alternatively, the examiners all dread the situation where a candidate answers 'I don't know' to all the initial questions, leaving the rest of the viva with nothing to talk about. Those bright stars who are up for prizes can expect to be asked extra questions which other candidates have only encountered in their worst nightmares. Most vivas consist of three basic questions, and you should aim to get through these in the 15 minutes. You may be asked four topics if you proceed 'at pace' through the first three.

Upon entering the hall, the candidates are told the letter of their allotted station where there will be two examiners; each viva is split into two equal halves by a bell, with alternate examiners conducting each half. Both examiners mark you in each part of the viva.

The vivas are split as follows:

• Clinical anaesthesia (15 minutes), and equipment and safety, physics and clinical measurement (15 minutes)
• Physiology including biochemistry (15 minutes) and pharmacology (15 minutes)

Candidates may be shown photographs, diagrams, equipment and so on, but the whole viva is essentially a series of topics/questions and answers. The emphasis on basic safety is reinforced by inclusion of a 'critical incident' in the clinical section for each candidate to discuss.

MARKING

In the past the vivas were prone to marking inconsistencies. For example, examiners' judgements of a candidate were sometimes influenced by their own values and it was possible that one candidate's performance could affect that of the following candidate. To eliminate this potential bias the vivas and OSCEs are structured. The questions that must be asked are in the sheet in front of the examiner and he/she cannot deviate in the questioning from them.

The same basic marking scheme as previously mentioned in

Chapter 1 (0: no show; 1: poor fail; 1+: fail; 2: pass; 2+: outstanding) is used in the vivas. Each examiner scores the candidate independently on the mark sheet before the two marks
are compared. Each also notes down the topics discussed
whilst the other examiner is conducting the viva so that both
examiners can run through the candidate's performance
together at the end of the viva. If the examiners' original
marks disagree, this process may help them agree on a final
mark. Reasons for a 1 or 1+ must be recorded on the examiners' marking sheet. At the examiners' meeting after the vivas
any inconsistencies are discussed (e.g. one candidate who
shines through all other parts but fails miserably in one viva)
and any score of 1 is also discussed. Last-minute decisions on
a particular candidate's performance may be taken although
this is apparently unusual.

TECHNIQUE

There are three areas to tackle when preparing for the vivas:

1. Basic appearance and behaviour
2. Knowledge
3. Strategies for handling the questions

1. Appearance and behaviour

Everyone says it and they're right. Look tidy, avoid loud
clothes and bold colours, and get that haircut that you have
been planning for the last few weeks. Your aim is to impress
the examiners with your tidiness, politeness and general professional bearing, not your terrible dress sense. You also need
to apply some thought to your body language. It's quite
amazing when observing the examination, just how often a
candidate shuffles up, slumps into the chair with a sigh and
gets the whole business off to a bad start. Saying 'Oh No!' and
flopping over the table after being asked the first question
looks terrible and makes a lasting impression. Watch how
others sit and move when they answer questions in practice

vivas, making mental notes about what you think is good and what is bad. Stand or sit in front of the mirror and try to look happy and confident, yet humble. Defensive postures typically involve crossed limbs; try to avoid sitting hunched over with your arms tightly crossed across your chest. Try also to avoid aggressive behaviour such as pointing at the examiners or striking the table (or the examiner with a John Prescott left hook!) to emphasize a point and try not to let your hands form a fist. Also, don't slouch in the chair with your head propped up on your hand(s). Try to assume a relaxed non-threatening posture by sitting upright with your hands gently clasped in your lap or on the table in front of you. Keeping your palms facing upwards suggests openness and is generally a good thing if you move your hands. Watch also how you gesticulate and move when you talk - the examiners will appreciate the odd sign that you are awake and you can show them you are listening to them by nodding occasionally, but they do not want to be faced with a windmill-like display of frantic arm waving. Other things to be avoided include putting your hands to your mouth or face (suggests you are not speaking the truth!), moving your eyes all over the place when you talk (suggests you are shifty!) and scratching various parts of your anatomy (suggests you have scabies!). Speak directly to the examiner who is questioning you.

When the examiners speak, you must try to look attentive (leaning forward slightly gives an air of keenness) and when you answer, try to speak slowly and clearly. Like everything else you're reading, this is easy to say but difficult to do, hence the importance of practising in front of the mirror and in front of other people. Try to adopt the same posture as the person you are facing. This instantly puts the other person at ease.

Making eye contact is crucial to good communication, but it can be difficult to stare your examiners in the face when you feel so intimidated. A good trick is to stare at a point on the examiners' forehead when answering a question - they will not be able to tell that you are not looking directly at their eyes.

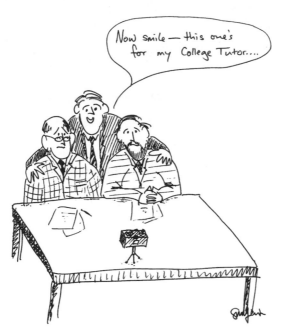

A number of courses use videos to illustrate deficiencies in candidates' presentation and its oftcn a shock to see just how badly you present yourself when seen from someone else's perspective. Get your colleagues to comment on your performance. Spouses and partners are particularly good at this sort of constructive criticism and may leap at the chance to offer corrective advice.

When speaking try to vary your tone occasionally so that you don't drone on in a monotone. This definitely requires practice, since it feels quite odd at first. Once again, the only way to do it is to say the same couple of sentences again and again, trying out different ways of varying your voice until it sounds satisfactory. You do need to be alone for this; the car is a particularly good place if you drive to work since you can devote every journey to a spot of voice practice. You must also practise speaking without using those really irritating clichés such as 'OK', 'right', 'you know', 'basically', 'at the end of the day', 'we was robbed, Brian' and so on.

2. Knowledge

The knowledge you have acquired for passing the MCQ examination will stand you in good stead for answering the vivas. However, this part of the examination will also test how you *apply* your factual knowledge.

3. Handling the questions

We cannot overemphasize the importance of listening to the question. It's amazing how often this isn't done; if the examiner asks 'Tell me how you would anaesthetize a patient with diabetes for amputation of a leg', don't launch straight into a discourse on invasive monitoring, even though it may come up in the ensuing discussion and you may know all about it. It may be helpful to start any answer with a brief statement setting the scene, such as 'My main concerns in this case would be the effect of diabetes on the various body systems; the perioperative control of the blood sugar; and the fact that this patient needs an amputation'. This kind of preliminary statement achieves two aims: it tells the examiners that you have this question sorted out in your mind in case you run out of time later. It also helps you set the scene for yourself, giving you a few extra microseconds to get your thoughts in order. Try this doing this each time you practise questions.

The rest of your answer should be as logical and structured as you can make it. Practise thinking in terms of subject headings, listing them to yourself first, then going back over each point in detail. For example, a general question on difficult intubation could be answered thus: 'Difficult intubation is an uncommon but serious problem in anaesthetic practice, the main concerns being (i) definition, (ii) preoperative prediction (iii) management of the acute unexpected case and (iv) management of the known case'. You can then address these points in turn. It can be difficult to come out with this kind of structured answer afresh, hence the importance of practising viva questions and observing others.

One problem of the structured answer is when there is more

than one possible approach, e.g. answering a question about hypotension during anaesthesia. This could be answered according to causes: 'Since MAP = CO × SVR, then hypotension could result from a decrease in CO or in SVR. Since CO = SV × HR, a fall in CO could in turn result from a decrease in either of these. Causes of reduced SV include decreased venous return, decreased myocardial contractility'. However, the same question could also be answered according to management: 'The first step would be to give IV fluids, increase the FIO_2 and quickly scan the surgical field for increased bleeding or excessive force on the retractors, I would also scan the patient generally for chest expansion, colour and capillary refill and look at the monitors, especially pulse oximeter, capnograph'. It can be difficult sometimes to know which approach is best for any particular question and there may not always be an obvious clue in the question's wording. The approach you use may depend on the context (e.g. clinical or pharmacological) in which the question is answered. If you really are unsure what emphasis is required, one strategy is actually to ask the examiners: 'Would you like me to go through the causes first and then discuss management, or describe what I would actually do in practice?'.

Don't pepper your answers with references - although it's all right to mention the odd paper this won't be on the examiners' list of required topics and they're likely to know the literature better than you do.

Also, don't try to steer the viva. If the examiner asks about difficult intubation, you are unlikely to be able to manipulate the conversation around to the pharmacology of antiemetics and the examiners will get cross if you drift from the subject asked, given the list of topics and required points in front of them. They won't mind being led a little, though, if that makes the viva flow more smoothly. One way of making it all flow better is to pre-empt the examiner's next question. It can be quite irritating for an examiner constantly to have to ask for little snippets of your answer. Thus, if you are asked 'What investigation would you request for a patient with ischaemic heart disease undergoing surgery', don't answer 'ECG, chest

X-ray, haemoglobin'. Instead, say 'First, I would request an ECG looking for rhythm abnormalities, signs of ischaemia such as T wave depression, T wave inversion, Q waves or conduction defects. I would also ask for a chest X-ray to look for signs of cardiac failure'.

Something that may easily happen during a viva is that your mind goes absolutely blank, usually just after you have been asked a question. This is quite acceptable so long as you explain to the examiners that your mind has gone blank and would they mind repeating the question, rather than sitting there with your mouth opening and closing like a goldfish. A similar situation is when you say the first thing that comes into your mind even though it's not quite appropriate for the occasion (e.g. in response to the question 'How would you induce anaesthesia in a patient with epilepsy', giving the answer 'Not ketamine'. We have heard the question 'What drugs do you give to raise blood pressure' being answered by 'Pancuronium'. Pancuronium does indeed cause a tachycardia, but is not our first choice for raising blood pressure! This would lead to a high mortality in the non-anaesthetized population!). It's probably best to follow a gaffe like this with an immediate apology and a request to start again, which will probably be granted. Another thing you should do if you really have no idea about the answer to a question is to come clean and own up that you don't know, rather than go through the humiliating and tiresome process of having your ignorance dragged out of you. It also gives you a chance to redeem yourself later. Alternatively, if you think your answer is reasonable, then stick to your guns if the examiner leans on you a little – you'll impress with your conviction and standing up to pressure, so long as you are prepared to back down if the examiner really presses hard.

One other thing – don't be put off if the examiners suddenly change the subject when you're in mid-flow. This can be quite distracting but it's usually a reflection of the examiners' requirement for covering all the topics on their list.

Viva Examination A

VIVA I (PHARMACOLOGY/PHYSIOLOGY)

EXAMINER I – PHARMACOLOGY

Q1. Discuss the factors that influence the transfer of drugs across the placenta.

The placental barrier is composed of a single layer of chorion (placenta) in contact with the fetal endothelial cells. This barrier behaves like a lipid membrane similar to the blood-brain barrier.

Factors which influence the transfer of drugs include:

- Lipid solubility – small lipid soluble drugs pass easily
- Degree of ionization – only unionized drugs pass easily, large ionized drugs do not cross. The pH of the maternal blood may alter the degree of ionization
- Molecular weight of the drug – small molecules (<600 daltons) pass easily
- Maternal-fetal concentration gradient
- Protein binding – protein-bound drugs are 'held' in the maternal blood; low plasma proteins (e.g. pre-eclampsia) will increase the amount of free drug and increase placental transfer
- Placental surface area – will influence the area available for diffusion
- Maternal placental blood flow which influences the amount of drug available for transfer

Which drugs used during general anaesthesia for caesarean section cross the placenta and what are the potential problems for the neonate?

Classify the answer to this question in a logical manner or you may omit an important group of drugs in the stress of the viva. Describe them in the sequence they are given during a GA section.

- *Induction agent.* Thiopentone is commonly used. It is a highly lipid soluble weak acid, at plasma pH 61% is unionized and 75% is protein-bound. It readily crosses the placenta.

- *Inhalational anaesthetic agents.* These are small highly lipid soluble molecules which cross the placenta within 1 min. Nitrous oxide crosses the placenta easily and may cause diffusion hypoxia in the neonate.
- *Muscle relaxants.* These are large highly polarized molecules and therefore do not cross the placenta and pose no clinical problems to the neonate.
- *Analgesics.* All opioids cross the placenta in significant amounts. Of the opioids commonly used, pethidine is only 50% protein-bound and has a large placental transfer, the maximum occurring 2-3 h after an intramuscular injection. This is the time of greatest risk of respiratory depression in the fetus. The half-life of pethidine and norpethidine are much longer in the fetus. Morphine is less lipid soluble but because of its poor protein binding there is a greater proportion of free drug which readily crosses the placenta. Fentanyl is very lipid soluble and crosses the placenta rapidly.
- *Anticholinergics.* Glycopyrrolate being polarized does not cross the placenta unlike atropine and hyoscine which readily cross.
- *Vasoactive drugs.* Sympathomimetics such as ephedrine are commonly used during regional anaesthesia for caesarean section. It is a naturally occurring amine and readily crosses the placenta. Hydrallazine, a commonly used hypotensive agent in pre-eclampsia, has a high degree of protein binding which reduces placental transfer. Many β-blockers are lipid soluble (e.g. propranolol, esmolol) and readily cross the placenta causing fetal bradycardias.

Epidurals are commonly used to provide analgesia during labour. Is the fetus at risk from the local anaesthetic and/or opioid given by this route?

This question is really asking about systemic absorption of drugs from the epidural space.

For the fetus to be affected by drugs given into the epidural space they have to be absorbed into the systemic circulation prior to placental transfer. The epidural space is highly vascular with large venous plexuses. Bupivacaine and ropivacaine are commonly used and some systemic absorption is to be expected as they are highly lipid soluble. Placental transfer will be reduced due to the high degree of protein binding (around 95%). Fentanyl is the opioid commonly used in combination with local anaesthetic for epidural analgesia. Its high lipid solubility encourages systemic absorption from the epidural space. Approximately 80–90% of the drug is protein-bound and at plasma pH 91% of the drug is ionized. Both these factors reduce placental transfer.

Is there a significant clinical problem?

Local anaesthetics and opioids are commonly administered via the epidural route in labour, and although subtle effects have been observed in the fetus in research studies there appears to be no clinical problem in the vast majority of cases. Like many situations in anaesthesia one has to balance the advantages of superior analgesia with the risks of systemic absorption of drugs which may affect the fetus if they cross the placenta.

Related questions

- *Name the factors which influence drug transfer into breast milk?*
- *What advice would you give to a lactating mother about to undergo general anaesthesia for emergency surgery?*
- *Discuss teratogenicity. How are drugs screened for teratogenicity?*
- *Many drugs used in anaesthetic practice act on the brain and CNS, what factors influence passage of drugs across the blood-brain barrier?*

Q2. What are the properties of an ideal anaesthetic volatile agent?

There are many factors to be considered and these need classifying, they would normally be classified into the physical properties of the agent and the pharmacological and physiological effects it has on the patient.

I will discuss the physical properties of an ideal volatile agent before discussing the physiological and pharmacological effects on the patient.

The agent should be a stable liquid at room temperature and not decomposed by light. It should have a reasonably long shelf-life without the need for preservative. It should be noninflammable and non-corrosive if spilt. It should not breakdown in soda-lime. It should have a high saturated vapour pressure (SVP) so that vaporization occurs easily.

The agent should be non-pungent and non-irritant to the upper airway so that it may be used for gaseous induction when required. It should have a low blood/gas solubility to allow rapid changes in the level of anaesthesia. It should be potent so that anaesthesia may be achieved at low inspired concentrations to allow the co-administration of high concentrations of oxygen.

The agent should not produce adverse physiological effects. It should not sensitize the myocardium to catecholamines and should have minimal negative inotropic effects on cardiac contractility. It should not produce or enhance conduction delays/defects. The agent should be non-irritant to the airway and preferably have bronchodilator effects. It should produce rapid smooth onset of anaesthesia and be non-epileptogenic. It should have predictable EEG effects and be free of excitatory or involuntary movements. It should have minimal effects on cerebral vasodilatation and intracranial pressure.

It should be relatively inert having minimal metabolism and be unaffected by hepatic or renal failure. It should have no toxic metabolites and should not trigger malignant hyperpyrexia.

Which agent do you think approaches this ideal and which is furthest from it?
No agent fulfils *all* the criteria of an ideal agent. The agent that is nearest to the ideal is probably sevoflurane, although there have been some concerns regarding toxic breakdown products in soda lime. Halothane is far from ideal as it has a high blood/gas solubility, sensitizes the myocardium to cate-

cholamines, has a high level of metabolism to potentially toxic metabolites and the solution requires the addition of preservative.

What is the mechanism for halothane toxicity?

Halothane is metabolized by both oxidative and reductive pathways. One of the oxidative metabolites (trifluoroacetyl chloride) appears to bind to the hepatocyte cell membrane to form a hapten. Antibodies may be produced to this complex which is recognized as a foreign protein. At subsequent administration of halothane a severe immune-mediated inflammatory reaction may occur. This can lead to fulminant hepatic failure associated with a high mortality rate of greater than 50%.

Is there a diagnostic test for halothane toxicity?

A test exists for 'halothane antibodies'. This involves testing the patient's serum to see if antibodies are present which react to *in vitro* rabbit hepatocytes previously exposed to halothane *in vivo*. These antibodies are detected by an enzyme-linked immunosorbent assay (ELISA).

Now let us imagine that you are about to perform an inhalational induction on a patient. What factors influence how quickly the patient becomes anaesthetized?

Anaesthesia occurs once a certain partial pressure is reached in the lungs which is in equilibrium with the brain. You need to think about factors bringing the agent to the lungs and those taking it away.

The patient becomes unconscious when the necessary partial pressure is achieved in the lungs which is in equilibrium with the brain compartment.

Factors which increase the rate at which this partial pressure is achieved include factors bringing the volatile agent to the lungs. This will be dependent on:

- The inspired concentration of the volatile agent, provided that this concentration is not irritant to the airway which

would result in coughing and breath-holding which would delay uptake
- The respiratory rate and tidal volume (= minute volume)

The increase in partial pressure will be slowed by factors removing the volatile agent from the lungs including
- Cardiac output (a high cardiac output will carry the volatile agent away from the lungs and vice versa)
- The blood/gas solubility which affects the amount of volatile agent removed per unit volume of blood.

Can you illustrate the effect of blood/gas solubility on the uptake of volatile agent?
This can be illustrated by drawing a graph of the ratio of fractional alveolar concentration of the agent/fractional inspired concentration of volatile agent against time. Equilibration occurs when this ratio approaches 1.

Draw a graph similar to that in Figure 3.1 – don't forget to label the axes.

Agents (e.g. N_2O and desflurane) with the lowest blood gas solubility of about 0.4 rapidly reach equilibrium within 15–20 min. Isoflurane and enflurane have intermediate blood gas solubilities of 1.4 and 1.8, respectively. Halothane has the highest blood/gas

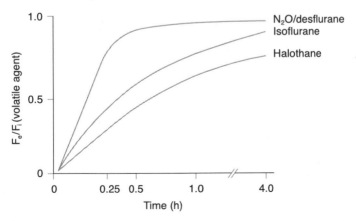

Figure 3.1 Uptake (or wash-in) curves of volatile agents.

solubility (2.3) of the agents currently available and equilibrium takes several hours to achieve. (In theory it never reaches equilibrium because of the high rate of metabolism.)

Q3. Non-steroidal anti-inflammatory drugs (NSAIDs) are commonly used as analgesics. How do NSAIDs work?

NSAIDs inhibit cyclo-oxygenase and thus reduce the production of prostaglandins along the arachidonic acid pathway. (*You may offer to draw the pathway.*)

How does this produce an analgesic action?
Prostaglandins are released during the inflammatory response to tissue trauma. These local prostaglandins increase the sensitivity of the peripheral nociceptor to noxious stimuli and an increase in nociceptive impulses results. NSAIDs also have central analgesic actions but the mechanism of this is unclear.

What are the side effects of the NSAIDs and how are these related to their pharmacodynamic actions?
In the *respiratory system* bronchospasm may be induced. This may be particularly severe in patients with aspirin induced bronchospasm.
   Platelet function is adversely affected by NSAIDs. This is due to inhibition of both thromboxane (pro-coagulant) production in the platelets and prostacyclin (anticoagulant) production in the vascular endothelial wall. As platelets are unable to regenerate cyclo-oxygenase the balance shifts, prostacyclin predominates and platelet adhesion is reduced.
   In the *GI tract* NSAIDs inhibit prostaglandin production which has a cytoprotective action in the gastric mucosa. Mucosal blood flow is also modified. This increases the risk of mucosal bleeding and in combination with reduced platelet adhesion can result in severe GI haemorrhage.
   In the *kidney*, a proportion of renal blood flow (RBF) is 'prostaglandin dependent'. This dependence is minimal in normal kidneys but becomes more significant when RBF is

compromised. In these situations reduced prostaglandin synthesis results in a reduction of RBF which may be enough to precipitate acute renal failure in susceptible patients. Patients who are most at risk include those with diabetes, congestive cardiac failure, hypertensives and trauma patients. Long term NSAID consumption may result in irreversible analgesic nephropathy due to direct toxic cellular damage.

What methods are available to reduce the side effects of NSAIDs?
Remember the basics before jumping to COX$_2$ inhibitors.

- Take a careful drug history, i.e. previous exposure and any problems, aspirin induced asthma, history of GI ulceration/bleeding
- Avoid high-risk groups who are prone to complications such as the elderly, diabetics and trauma patients
- Co-administration of prostaglandin analogues such as misoprostol for gastric mucosal cytoprotection
- Use COX$_2$ inhibitors

What is the rationale for using COX$_2$ inhibitors?
It has been shown that two iso-enzymes of cyclic-oxygenase exist. COX$_1$ regulates prostaglandin synthesis during normal physiological conditions. COX$_2$ is the iso-enzyme which is responsible for increased prostaglandin production during the inflammatory response. It is suggested that if COX$_2$ could be selectively inhibited, then the physiological role of prostaglandins could continue and side effects reduced compared to non-selective inhibitors.

Can you name a NSAID which is selective for COX$_2$ and is it associated with less side effects?
The majority of NSAIDs are non-selective for cyclo-oxygenase. During the year 2000 COX$_2$ selective drugs were introduced in the UK, an example being celoxib. Once these drugs are used in large numbers in long-term everyday clinical use we will have a clearer picture of their efficacy and side-effect profile. Until then,

we have to rely on the limited information from the initial phase II and phase III clinical trials which have demonstrated some reduction in side effects without loss of efficacy.

EXAMINER 2 – PHYSIOLOGY

Q1. Physiologists use a spirometer to measure lung volumes. How does a spirometer work?

A spirometer usually consists of a light, floating bell which floats on water (Benedict Roth). The air within the bell is in continuity with a breathing tube, through which the subject inspires and expires. During expiration the exhaled gas from the subject passes into the space under the bell which rises. The opposite happens during inspiration. These movements are recorded by a pen attached to the bell producing a spirometer trace on moving paper.

Would you like to draw such a trace and describe the volumes and capacities that can be derived from it?

You should be able to draw a spirometer trace. Do not confuse it with a vitalograph trace which is a clinical tool. There are four volumes and four capacities to remember. Draw Figure 3.2.

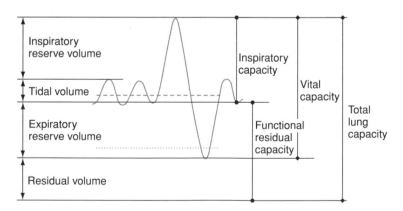

Figure 3.2 Spirometer traces illustrating lung volumes and capacities.

The tidal volume (TV) is the volume or air that is inspired and expired during normal respiration.

The residual volume (RV) is the volume of air remaining in the lung at the end of maximal expiration. This volume cannot be measured directly and has to be derived. The expiratory reserve volume (ERV) is the additional volume of air which can be maximally expired at the end of a normal tidal volume expiration. The functional residual capacity (FRC) is the combination of these two volumes and refers to the residual capacity of the lung at the end of a normal expiration.

The inspiratory reserve volume (IRV) is the additional volume of air inspired after a normal tidal volume inspiration up to maximal capacity. The total volume of air in the lung at this point is equal to the total lung capacity (TLC), which is the sum of the four lung volumes, i.e. TLC = IRV + TV + ERV + RV. The vital capacity (VC) is the volume of gas expired from maximal inspiration to maximal expiration. The inspiratory capacity (IC) is the volume of air inspired from expiration to maximum inspiration and is the combination of the tidal volume and inspiratory reserve volume.

What does the closing volume refer to?
The closing volume is the point, or lung volume, at which small airway closure begins. At this point, which occurs during expiration, the contracting lung volume is such that small airways are no longer held open by the surrounding expanded lung tissue and therefore collapse or 'close'.

Can you illustrate this on your spirometer drawing?
Draw dotted line on Figure 3.2.

The closing volume is normally less than the FRC and therefore occurs within the expiratory reserve volume and is outside the range of the tidal volume in a healthy patient.

Where would the closing volume occur in an obese patient?
The closing volume increases with obesity and the line moves up the trace and may impinge on the tidal volume. *(See dashed line Figure 3.2.)*

What is the significance of this to you as an anaesthetist?
Small airway closure results in distal alveolar collapse (atelectasis). These collapsed alveoli are unventilated yet remain perfused and a shunt occurs resulting in hypoxaemia. If the
closing volume occurs in the tidal volume range a proportion
of alveoli will be collapsed during normal respiration leading
to a persistent shunt and hypoxaemia and cyanosis at rest.
Additionally a much greater inspiratory effort is required to
reinflate these collapsed alveoli. Secretions may accumulate in
these alveoli predisposing to a chest infection.

**The functional residual capacity is also important to the anaes-
thetist. How would you measure this?**
The functional residual capacity (FRC) cannot be measured
directly as it is impossible to measure the residual volume of
the lung. The functional residual capacity has to be derived
from indirect measurements which estimate this volume by a
gas dilution method. Helium is used as this is relatively insoluble in blood, no helium is lost from the system and the
amount of helium (concentration multiplied by volume) is the
same at the beginning and at end the end of the experiment. A
spirometer (volume V_1) is filled with a concentration of helium
(C_1) in oxygen. The subject then breathes through the system
to allow equilibration of helium (C_2) in the volume of the system plus the subject's lungs (V_2). This larger volume (V_2) is
equal to $V_1 + \text{FRC}$.

Since $\quad C_1 V_1 = C_2 V_2$

and $\quad V_2 = (V_1 + \text{FRC})$ it is possible to derive the FRC
as follows

$$C_1 V_1 = C_2(V_1 + \text{FRC})$$
$$= C_2 V_1 + C_2 \text{FRC}$$

$$C_1 V_1 - C_2 V_1 = C_2 \text{FRC}$$
$$V_1(C_1 - C_2)/C_2 = \text{FRC}$$

Q2. What structure is responsible for the transmission of a motor nerve impulse from the nerve to a skeletal muscle fibre?

Once you have stated the structure, give a simple description.

This occurs at the motor end plate. This is a specialized area where the terminal of the motor fibre is in close proximity with the cell membrane of the muscle fibre. The two components are separated by a synaptic cleft.

Can you draw the structure?

You should be able to draw a diagram of this structure (see Figure 3.3). You should include and label the following structures.

- *The* motor neurone axon *(covered by a myelin sheath) ending in*
- *The* motor axon terminal button *which contains*
- Acetylcholine vesicles

The motor end plate membrane should be in close proximity to

- *The* post-synaptic muscle membrane *(sarcolemma) which is a folded membrane*
- *The* acetylcholine receptors *are located on this membrane*
- *The enzyme* acetylcholinesterase *is also located in the folds*
- *The two membranes are separated by the* synaptic cleft

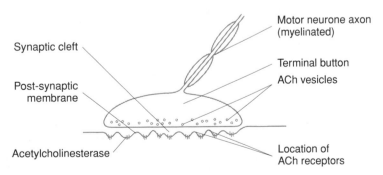

Figure 3.3 Structure of the neuro-muscular junction.

How does the impulse pass from nerve to muscle?
The impulse is transmitted from nerve to muscle by the release of acetylcholine (ACh) which diffuses across the synaptic cleft to depolarize the post-junctional muscle cell membrane. ACh is released when the nerve action potential travelling along the motor axon reaches the motor end plate. The local depolarization at the end-plate results in an influx of calcium into the nerve terminal which facilitates the movement of ACh vesicles towards the synaptic membrane. When the membranes of the two structures fuse, ACh is released. Each nerve action potential releases a set quantity of acetylcholine into the synaptic cleft. This 'quanta' of ACh diffuses across the synaptic cleft and binds to the ACh receptors on the post-synaptic membrane and triggers cell depolarization.

What is the structure of the acetylcholine receptor?
Remember the key words: transmembrane, ligand gated ion channel.

The ACh receptor is a transmembrane, ligand gated ion channel. It comprises of five protein subunits (2α, β, γ and δ) arranged in a cylinder surrounding an ion channel which spans the cell membrane. The ACh binding sites are located on the extracellular surface of the two α subunits.

What happens when acetylcholine binds to the receptor?
When acetylcholine binds to the receptors on the α subunits, a conformational change takes place in the protein subunits. The central ion channel opens allowing sodium ions to diffuse into the cell down an electrochemical gradient. Diffusion of positive sodium ions into the muscle cell raises the membrane potential from -70 mV towards the threshold for generation of a muscle action potential. Once this threshold is reached the subsequent action potential travels along the muscle cell membrane in a similar fashion to the passage along a nerve terminal. This potential is called the end-plate potential.

How does this result in muscle contraction?

In other words describe excitation-contraction coupling.

Excitation-contraction coupling describes the link between the muscle cell membrane depolarizing and contraction of the myofibrils. The muscle cell depolarization spreads over the surface membrane (sarcolemma) and down into the cell via the T tubules. These tubules are in close contact with the sarcoplasmic reticulum which networks intracellularly in close contact with the myofilaments. The sarcoplasmic reticulum contains high concentrations of calcium. The spreading wave of depolarization results in release of this calcium into the myoplasm adjacent to the myofilaments. The myofilaments comprise of actin and myosin filaments which are the contractile mechanism of the myofibril. The calcium binds to troponin C on the actin filament triggering a conformational change in which active sites on the actin myofilament form 'cross-bridges' between the actin and myosin filaments. These cross-bridges then 'walk along' or ratchet causing contraction of the myofibril.

What is the resting concentration of calcium in the muscle cell?

This is a factual question that you will either know or not know. Do not waste time pondering such questions that may come up in the course of viva questions. It is important to move on to other parts of the question that you can answer to continue scoring points. If you do not know you can either make an educated guess or say 'I am sorry I can't recall this at the moment may I come back to this question later?'. You should only use this tactic once with each set of examiners and it should not be employed for answers where you really should know the answer!

The resting concentration of Ca^{2+} is 10^{-7} to 10^{-8} mmol/l.

Do you know what it changes to during contraction?

(See above)

It rises to 10^{-5} mmol/l during contraction.

Once the myofibril has contracted, how does the cell prepare for further contractions?
Once depolarization occurs the resting membrane potential is restored by membrane Na^+/K^+ pumps which restore ion balance and repolarize the cell. The calcium released from the sarcoplasmic reticulum during excitation-contraction coupling is rapidly pumped back by an energy requiring Ca^{2+} pump. When the intracellular calcium concentration decreases, the cross-links between the actin and myosin break down and the myofilaments slide apart as the myofibril relaxes.

What happens to the acetylcholine once it has bound to the receptor?
Once the ion channel opens and depolarization occurs, the ACh molecule dissociates from the binding sites on the receptors into the synaptic cleft. Acetylcholinesterase which is located in the troughs of the folded post-junctional membrane, rapidly hydrolyses the ACh into acetate and choline. Much of this released choline is transported back into the nerve ending by a Na^+-dependent active pump for resynthesis.

Q3. Our surgical colleagues are performing increasing amounts of laparoscopic surgery, what are the physiological effects of a pneumoperitoneum?

This is another example of a question which requires classification so that you do not omit parts of the answer – answer the question in physiological systems. This question may branch off into other areas of physiology, the anaesthetic implications of these changes may be asked in the clinical viva. Keep talking until the examiner interrupts.

The physiological effects of a pneumoperitoneum are related to the physical effect of increased pressure within the abdominal cavity and the physiological effects of the gas (usually CO_2) used.

Outline the changes secondary to the physical effect of the gas
In the *cardiovascular system* (CVS), the increased intraperitoneal pressure increases the external pressure on the inferior vena cava which reduces the venous return to the right atrium. This reduction in venous return results in a drop in right atrial and right ventricular filling pressures. Right-sided end-diastolic volumes fall with a resultant drop in stroke volume. This in turn results in a decrease in blood return to the left side of the heart causing a fall in stroke volume and cardiac output. (Since CO = SV × HR, where CO = cardiac output, SV = stroke volume and HR = heart rate.) Reflex compensatory mechanisms will result to counter the fall in cardiac output. As the cardiac output falls there will be a drop in blood pressure due to the relationship; BP = CO × SVR (where BP = blood pressure and SVR = systemic vascular resistance). This drop in BP triggers a baroreceptor response.

What are baroreceptors?
The baroreceptors are stretch receptors located in the wall of the carotid artery. The rate of firing is directly proportional to the wall pressure.

(Continue with your original answer now as it follows on.)

As the blood pressure falls the rate of nerve impulses in these inhibitory fibres falls and there is a reduction in inhibitory 'tone' to the sympathetic centre. This results in increased sympathetic discharge from the sympathetic centre, catecholamine levels rise causing an increase in heart rate and an increase in systemic vascular resistance.

Additionally, stretch receptors in the right atrium will detect less stretch as filling volumes fall. This causes a reduction in natriuretic hormone so that ultimately less sodium is excreted in the urine. This mechanism restores plasma volume and increases venous return.

In the *respiratory system* the increased intra-abdominal pressure splints the diaphragm. This causes a reduction in the functional residual capacity (FRC) resulting in atelectasis and shunting in the collapsed alveoli. Diaphragmatic splinting also reduces the chest compliance causing a fall in tidal volume which will reduce the minute ventilation unless the respiratory rate were to increase. Any decrease in minute volume will result in an increase in arterial CO_2 tension.

In the *central nervous system* an increase in cerebral blood flow (CBF) and intracranial pressure (ICP) may occur. These changes are secondary to increased arterial CO_2 and the resultant cerebral vasodilatation. Intracranial pressure would rise secondary to not only increased CBF but the increase in venous pressure that is associated with the Trendelenburg (head down) position.

In the *abdominal system* increased intraperitoneal pressure increases the external pressure on the stomach. This produces a rise in intragastric pressure and if this exceeds the overall barrier pressure at the lower oesophageal sphincter there will be an increased risk of regurgitation. As the cardiac output falls there is a reduction in splanchnic blood flow secondary to sympathetic mechanisms to preserve cardiac output.

In the *renal system* there will be a fall in renal blood flow secondary to the reduction in splanchnic blood flow. Glomerular filtration will fall. This is detected at the juxtaglomerular apparatus and renin is released. Renin converts angiotensinogen to angiotensin I which is further converted to angiotensin II as it passes through the lungs. These are potent vasoconstrictors which increase systemic vascular resistance to compensate for the decrease in renal perfusion pressure. Aldosterone release from the adrenal cortex is increased secondary to the fall in blood volume and increased renin/angiotensin release. The increase in aldosterone promotes salt (and water) retention by the kidneys in a compensatory mechanism to increase blood volume thus restoring cardiac output.

Why is carbon dioxide commonly used to produce the pneumoperitoneum?
CO_2 is readily available as a medical gas. It is a colourless gas which doesn't support combustion which is a necessary factor if diathermy is used. Additionally CO_2 is relatively soluble in

the blood so that if an inadvertent venous emboli occurred the CO_2 would rapidly dissolve.

What are the physiological effects of high arterial CO_2?

(This answer should be classified as above. At this point in the viva we would list the effects and wait for the examiner to ask you to expand on any point or the bell to ring!)

A high $PaCO_2$ causes a respiratory acidosis in the arterial blood. In the cardiovascular system (CVS) high arterial $PaCO_2$ results in an increase in sympathetic tone, this would manifest as a tachycardia, increased blood pressure and a full bounding pulse. In the respiratory system there would be increased respiratory drive leading to a rapid respiratory rate and high minute volumes in a spontaneously breathing subject. In the CNS increased $PaCO_2$ causes cerebral vasodilatation which may result in the awake patient complaining of headaches. A peripheral tremor may be present. If $PaCO_2$ levels continue to rise eventually CO_2 narcosis occurs.

What compensatory mechanism occurs in patients with chronic CO_2 retention?

Chronic CO_2 retention causes a respiratory acidosis. To maintain plasma pH the acid 'load' that cannot be excreted by the lungs has to be buffered in the blood by bicarbonate. The kidney compensates for this by increasing bicarbonate reabsorption in the proximal and distal tubules.

How does the kidney achieve this?

The polarized bicarbonate ions, filtered by the glomerulus, are not readily reabsorbed through the tubular cell membrane. The filtered HCO_3^- ions combine with H^+ ions secreted into the tubule lumen to form carbonic acid which dissociates into H_2O and CO_2. The CO_2 then readily diffuses into the tubule cell where intracellular carbonic anhydrase catalyses rehydration of CO_2 back to carbonic acid which then re-dissociates to H^+ (which is secreted back into the tubule to combine with more bicarbonate) and HCO_3^- which is reabsorbed into the blood. Overall there is a net excretion of acid and reabsorption of bicarbonate.

Thank you.
Thank you.

VIVA 2 (CLINICAL MEASUREMENT, PHYSICS AND CLINICAL)

EXAMINER 1 – CLINICAL MEASUREMENT/PHYSICS

Q1. What types of vaporizers are commonly used in anaesthetic practice?

(There are only two commonly used.)

Two types of vaporizers are commonly used; these are plenum vaporizers and drawover vaporizers.

Can you give an example of a plenum vaporizer?
The 'TEC' series are plenum vaporizers.

What are the basic features of a TEC vaporizer and how does it work?
A TEC vaporizer is a factory-calibrated, temperature-compensated plenum vaporizer. The vaporizer works under positive pressure so that the carrying gas (from the flow meters) is driven through it. Inside the vaporizer the gas is split into two pathways in which one pathway passes through the vaporizing chamber which contains the volatile agent and becomes saturated with vapour. In the other pathway the remaining gas flow passes through a bypass chamber where no vapour is added. The two gas pathways merge distally to produce a mixture containing the concentration of agent 'dialled up'. The relative amount of gas passing through each pathway is determined by the *splitting ratio* which depends on the concentration of agent selected and the temperature in the vaporizing chamber. As evaporation occurs from the volatile liquid, its temperature drops. The TEC vaporizer incorporates a large block of copper under the vaporization chamber which acts as a heat sink.

What features does the vaporizer have to ensure the correct concentration of volatile agent is delivered?
The vaporizer is calibrated for a single volatile agent only since the concentration delivered is dependent on the saturated

vapour pressure (SVP). Metal wicks inside the vaporizing chamber increase the surface area available for evaporation which ensures that the vapour above the liquid surface is saturated, i.e. at SVP. As evaporation occurs, the temperature drops, and since saturated vapour pressure is temperature dependent and the concentration of volatile agent is expressed as a partial pressure, the vaporizer must compensate for temperature to maintain a constant output. This is achieved with a bimetallic strip which increases the proportion of gas passing through the vaporizing chamber as the temperature drops.

Outline methods that other vaporizers employ to encourage vaporization?
The carrier gas may be bubbled through the volatile agent (Boyle's bottle).
Baffles may be used to ensure the carrier gas passes closely over the liquid level.
The volatile agent may be actively heated to increase the saturated vapour pressure (Desflurane vaporizer).

What safety features exist in TEC vaporizers?
The vaporizer is clearly labelled and colour coded for the volatile agent it is intended to deliver. A key filling mechanism ensures that the vaporizer can only be filled with the agent it is intended (and calibrated) for. The concentration dial requires a secondary ratchet button to be pressed to release the dial from zero so it cannot be opened accidentally. A mechanism exists to prevent the bypass chamber from contamination with volatile agent should the vaporizer be inadvertently tilted. Vaporizers in the TEC4 series and more recent versions have a 'Selactatec' mechanism which ensures that only one vaporizer can be open in machines where it is possible to have more than one vaporizer on the back bar.

What do you understand by the term saturated vapour pressure?
This is the partial pressure of a vapour in an enclosed chamber which is in equilibrium with the liquid from which it has evaporated. At this pressure an equal number of molecules are

entering the gas as those leaving it. The pressure is constant for a particular agent at a given temperature.

What happens if a small heating element is placed under a chamber filled with a volatile liquid?
Application of heat increases the energy of the molecules in the liquid and more molecules pass from the liquid to the vapour phase above the liquid. This increased movement of molecules out of the liquid increases the pressure of the vapour.

What happens if enough heat is supplied to make the liquid boil?
The vapour above the boiling liquid will be at 1 atm. It is not possible to raise the temperature of the liquid any further unless pressure is applied to the vapour above it.

Finally how do drawover vaporizers differ from plenum vaporizers?
Drawover vaporizers have a low resistance to gas flow. Carrier gas is 'drawn' through the vaporizer by the application of a negative pressure on the outflow limb (rather than positive pressure at the inspiratory limb as in plenum vaporizers). The most simple drawover vaporizers cannot be accurately calibrated as they are not temperature compensated and variations in flow (secondary to the patient's tidal volume) affect the time available for vaporization and therefore the carrier gas is not necessarily saturated as it passes through the vaporizer.

In what situations would you use a drawover vaporizer?
I would use these in a circle system, and they may be used in portable anaesthetic equipment for use 'in the field' where there is no compressed gas supply.

Q2. Describe methods available for detecting end-expiratory carbon dioxide.

In the hospital environment capnography is utilized, these may employ mainstream or side stream analysers. Single use devices employed by paramedics outside the hospital environment contain chemical indicators. In these devices, which attach over the end of the tracheal tube, a chemical indicator changes colour when CO_2 passes through it.

How does a capnograph work?
It utilizes infrared (IR) absorption using a spectrophotometer. CO_2 absorbs IR light as it contains two different atoms. A single frequency wavelength of IR is directed through a sampling chamber and light intensity measured. Energy absorption (dependent on CO_2 concentration) is compared with a similar beam passing through a reference chamber.

What is the difference between a side-stream and a mainstream analyser?
A side-stream analyser is commonly used in clinical practice. Sample gas is drawn from the respiratory gas stream via a side-port and pumped to the analysing chamber which is remote from the patient. The sampling chamber is less bulky. However water condensation from expired breath can affect the measurement. A long cycling time occurs due to the time taken to pump gas to the sampling chamber.

In a mainstream analyser the entire respiratory gases pass through the analyser which is located across the breathing system. The analyser is necessarily bulky and fragile. These are more suited to low flow circuits as no gas is removed from the system. The response time is more rapid.

What information may be obtained from the capnograph?
You may be asked to illustrate these or be given a trace and asked to categorize what is happening (Figure 3.4).

- It is used to confirm tracheal tube placement
- It is employed as an indicator/alarm that ventilation is occurring
- To measure end-expiratory CO_2 (and therefore institute an appropriate minute volume ventilation)
- To detect rebreathing

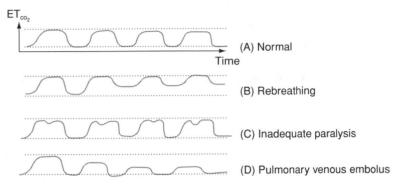

Figure 3.4 Sample capnograph traces.

- As an indirect (trend) indication of cardiac output
- It will indicate if a patient is making respiratory effort when neuromuscular paralysis is wearing off
- It will detect sudden drops of CO_2 output from the lung which occurs during air or fat embolus

Assume you are given the diagram shown in Figure 3.5. What does this capnograph trace tell you about the patient?

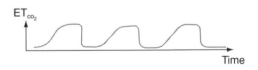

Figure 3.5 Capnograph trace for question 2.

Describe the trace first.

This capnograph shows a slow rising increase in CO_2 concentration during the expiratory phase (rather than the normal rapid upstroke and plateau seen in normal subjects). This indicates that the patient has airway disease, most commonly seen in patients with chronic obstructive airways disease.

How do you explain the sloping upstroke during expiration?
This indicates that the concentration of CO_2 in the expired gas is increasing during the expiratory phase of ventilation.

What causes the changing concentration of CO_2 in the expired breath?
This is caused by different alveoli being ventilated to different degrees during each ventilation. This is due to pathological processes in the distal airways causing variable changes in airway resistance coupled with variable compliance in the alveoli due to loss of elasticity in the surrounding lung tissue. In this situation there are a spectrum of alveoli being ventilated to different degrees. At one end of the spectrum there are 'fast' alveoli with elastic walls (low compliance) connected by airways with low resistance which receive preferential ventilation and therefore have a low CO_2 concentration. At the other end are 'slow' highly compliant alveoli connected to airways with a high resistance. These are poorly ventilated and gas moves in and out slowly such that CO_2 is not washed out and the concentration increases. The increasing contribution of these slow alveoli during the latter part of the expiratory cycle causes the concentration to rise.

Q3. Diathermy is commonly used during surgery. What are the different types of diathermy?

Diathermy may be unipolar or bipolar and the current applied may be coagulating or cutting.

What is the difference between unipolar and bipolar?
In unipolar diathermy a high frequency current passes through the body from the active (cutting or coagulation) electrode to a large neutral electrode stuck onto the surface of the patient's skin (base plate). The active electrode is usually a point which has a relatively small surface area; a high current density occurs causing a rapid rise in temperature resulting in coagulation or cutting in a localized tissue area.

In bipolar diathermy the current travels down one arm of

the forceps, passes through tissue in between the tips and completes the circuit by returning to the machine via the other arm.

What is the clinical difference between the two?
More energy can be delivered to the small active point in unipolar diathermy, allowing greater versatility to coagulate and cut tissue. In bipolar diathermy only a small amount of energy passes between the electrodes. This will be dissipated if there is heavy bleeding. Bipolar diathermy is used in situations where only a small area of diathermy is required such as neurosurgery or in situations where bleeding is reduced by the use a tourniquet.

What is the difference between cutting and coagulation modes?
The wave patterns of the applied current are different. A sinusoidal wave pattern is used for cutting and a damped waveform for coagulation.

What factors must be considered for the safe use of diathermy?
• The large plate must be in uniform contact with a large area of the patient's skin. If application is patchy a high current density may occur in small areas of contact resulting in a burn.
• If any other part of the patient touches metal (e.g. a lithotomy pole), a further potential route for current to pass is established if the table is earthed. A burn can result in the area of contact.
• When not in use, the active electrode/diathermy point should be kept in an insulated quiver to prevent burns if the diathermy were inadvertently activated whilst the point was lying against the patient's skin.
• Sparks from the diathermy may ignite flammable substances such as alcoholic skin preparations which may pool under the drapes or under the patient.
• If the base plate becomes disconnected, current will attempt to travel to earth via any point. If this area is small, high current density may result in a burn.

- If the patient has a pacemaker, the diathermy current may pass through the pacing wire and cause a burn at the tip. This may alter the pacing threshold and failure of the pacemaker to 'capture'.
- Diathermy currents may change the programming mode of complex programmable pacemaker units.

What precautions would you take in patients with a permanent pacemaker in situ?
I would try to persuade the surgeon to avoid the use of diathermy if at all possible. If diathermy is required, bipolar should be used rather than unipolar if sufficient. If unipolar diathermy is deemed necessary, the current path (from active to neutral electrodes) should not pass through the pacing unit or traverse the pacing wire.

I would ensure that a magnet is available in theatre. By placing this over a programmable pacing unit, it converts or reprogrammes the pacemakers to a fixed pacing mode in the event of failure due to programme interference. I would also consider referring the patient to the cardiologist so that a programmable pacemaker could be temporarily converted to a fixed mode.

EXAMINER 2 – CLINICAL TOPICS

Q1. An 81–year-old lady is found on the floor at home with pain in the hip. She is added to your evening emergency list for a hemiarthroplasty. What is your initial management?

Most candidates would start with 'I would go to the ward and take a full history and examine the patient'. You will look much more competent if you started with...

This patient needs a careful preoperative assessment, in addition to a routine anaesthetic history I would be particularly like to know:

- How the patient sustained the injury, which would ascertain

whether the patient had a simple trip or fall or a blackout
suggesting a medical cause for a fall
- How long the patient was on the floor before being found
which may give an indication of the possibility of dehydration and hypothermia
- Whether there were any other injuries such as a head injury
- How active the patient normally is, giving an indication of
exercise tolerance and whether the patient is confused
(which may rule out regional anaesthesia)

I would examine her paying particular attention to the
cardiorespiratory system and looking for signs of dehydration
(*you may be asked to expand this . . . talk about the difficulties
of these signs*), other injuries and evidence of confusion.

I would review investigations looking for the haemoglobin
result (which may be spuriously high in the presence of dehydration), electrolyte abnormalities particularly if the patient is
on diuretics, the ECG for arrhythmias and the CXR for
evidence of pneumonia or cardiac failure.

(*NB: Whenever you mention investigations you should always
mention the reason for doing it, or what you are looking for – as
in the answer above. Avoid listing investigations, in a reflex manner, if there is no reason for doing them.*)

**Examination of the patient reveals some pitting oedema of the
legs, a raised JVP, some fine inspiratory crackles at the lung
bases and a quiet systolic ejection murmur. What is your management now?**
These signs suggest cardiac failure (biventricular). The significance of the murmur needs to be established. The commonest
cause of this murmur in the elderly would be aortic sclerosis,
but significant aortic stenosis must be excluded. Signs sugges-
tive of significant aortic stenosis include a slow rising pulse, a
low systolic BP with a narrow pulse pressure, left ventricular
hypertrophy with or without signs of left ventricular failure.
The most relevant investigation would be an echocardiogram
which would give further information on LV function and

valve defects. A cardiology review would be useful to optimize treatment of her cardiac failure.

What would be the significance if her ECG revealed right bundle branch block (RBBB) and left axis deviation (LAD)?
This indicates a bifascicular block in which two out of the three main conductive fascicles are non-functioning. There is a significant risk of this block progressing to complete heart block. Asymptomatic bifascicular block would not necessarily be an indication for temporary pacing but if the patient were having blackouts (which could be the cause of her fall) one must consider the need for temporary pacing during the perioperative period. The advice of the cardiologist may be useful as they are likely to be the doctors inserting the pacing wire.

After 24 h of medical treatment, the patient's condition has improved and is deemed fit for surgery. What are your options for anaesthetic management for repair of fractured neck of femur?
One must choose between a general anaesthetic technique and a regional technique. If a regional technique is selected this could be performed by spinal or epidural techniques. If a general anaesthetic technique is selected, this may be a general anaesthetic alone with opioid analgesia or a combined GA/regional technique.

Which anaesthetic technique would you choose for the above patient?

At points in the viva you may be asked to decide between local, regional or general anaesthetic techniques. There isn't necessarily a right or wrong answer to such questions. The examiners expect you to reason the advantages over the disadvantages of the technique you chose...

Since the above patient presented with an element of cardiac failure I would proceed with a regional technique as this would reduce the afterload on the left ventricle. Before proceeding with this technique it would be important to exclude aortic stenosis and ensure the patient is cooperative and can lie flat for the duration of surgery. An epidural may be difficult to site in this age group, due to arthritic changes in the back. I would therefore elect to employ a spinal technique.

How would you perform this?
Assuming the patient consents to a regional technique she should be fasted as for a general anaesthetic. All equipment should be checked and necessary drugs, particularly vasopressors such as ephedrine, drawn up in labelled syringes. Standard monitoring should be attached and intravenous access secured with a wide-bore cannula placed under LA. Ideally one would preload a patient with 500–1000 ml of crystalloid before a spinal anaesthetic. This patient has a history of cardiac failure and therefore a cautious approach should be taken with fluid management including the use of vasopressor to treat hypotension rather than large fluid loads. The patient should be positioned either sitting or in a lateral position and the lumbar spaces identified. Using an aseptic technique *(expand if asked)* the patient's skin is disinfected and landmarks identified. The skin may be anaesthetized with local anaesthetic. I would use a relatively narrow bore 'pencil-tip' spinal needle (such as a 22 gauge) to locate CSF. Fine spinal needles may bend in arthritic backs. Once CSF is seen clearly in the hub of the spinal needle, 2–2.5 ml of local anaesthetic such as 0.5% bupivacaine may be injected. To achieve a unilateral block 'heavy' bupivacaine may be selected and the patient turned into a lateral position with the fractured leg in a dependent position (this may be difficult if the patient is in pain). Before proceeding to surgery the level of the block should be confirmed.

Surgery is progressing well until shortly after insertion of the prosthesis when the patient becomes bradycardic and hypotensive. What are the possible causes?
The most likely causes at this point would be:

1. Reaction to the cement
2. An ascending local anaesthetic block

3. An anaesthetic cause such as hypoxia from incorrect oxygen delivery or airway problems
4. A primary cardiac cause

How would you treat this event?
The heart rate should be increased since this will increase cardiac output and blood pressure, glycopyrrolate would be a suitable anticholinergic. A vasopressor should be employed to raise the systemic vascular resistance, ephedrine would be appropriate since its beta-adrenoceptor effects will have mild positive inotropic effects. The intravenous infusion may be increased cautiously (taking into account her past medical history of left ventricular failure) and 100% oxygen given by face mask. Blood pressure measurements should be measured frequently.

Tips/Hints

Remember the principles of any local anaesthetic block:

• *Contraindications*
• *Patient consent/cooperation*
• *Preparation – NBM, assistant, equipment, resuscitation, monitoring*
• *Performing – asepsis, position, LA agent/concentration/volume, needle, landmarks*
• *Checking level and adequacy of the block*
• *Complications – general (every block), specific, associated with the local anaesthetic.*

Q2. Anaesthetists commonly administer blood transfusions to their patients, what are the complications of blood transfusion?

There are many side effects, therefore you should classify these so that you don't miss any major ones out.

The complications of blood transfusion can be classified into immediate and delayed.
    The immediate side effects include:

- Immune-mediated blood transfusion reactions may occur to any blood cell component.
  - The most serious is major ABO mismatch which has a mortality of up to 10%. Natural IgM antibodies in the recipients blood lyse donor red cells triggering shock, DIC and haemoglobinuria. This usually occurs due to the wrong blood being given to the wrong patient.
  - Less serious reactions may occur to minor red cell antigens such as Kell and Duffy which result in febrile reactions followed by haemolysis over several days and recurrence of anaemia.
  - White cell reactions caused by acquired (previous transfusion) recipient antibodies reacting with antigens on donor white cells causing a mild febrile reaction.
  - Reaction to platelets occurs in patients requiring repeated platelet transfusions. Destruction of platelets results in failure of transfusion.
- Volume overload, is a common problem (often overlooked) especially in the elderly.
- Dilution of platelets and plasma clotting factors will result in a coagulopathy + bleeding disorders (especially in massive transfusion).
- Hypothermia.
- Hyperkalaemia (from K^+ which has leaked out of the stored RBCs).
- Citrate toxicity.
- Acute lung injury (due to microemboli).
- Immune modulation/suppression.

Delayed side effects include:

- Transmission of infection.
  - Viral, i.e. HIV, HBV, HCV, Epstein-Barr virus, cytomegalovirus.
  - Bacterial – this is rare as bacteraemic donors are seldom well enough to donate blood.
  - Parasitic, e.g. malaria.
  - Prion (new variant Creutzfeldt-Jakob disease).
- Rhesus incompatibility: Rhesus-negative patients given

Rhesus-positive blood develop acquired IgG antibodies which react with subsequent transfusions of Rhesus-positive blood to cause haemolysis. The IgG antibodies can cross the placenta to cause *haemolytic disease of the newborn* in Rhesus-negative babies.

• Iron overload which is a particular problem in patients requiring repeated transfusions over a number of years such as thalassaemia major.

Bearing in mind the complications you have mentioned what blood conservation strategies are available to reduce the need for allogenic blood transfusion?

These methods can be divided into preoperative and peroperative.

In preoperative autologous blood donation patients 'donate' units of blood in the weeks prior to surgery for retransfusion during surgery eliminating the risk of infection and immune reaction.

Preoperative erythropoietin may be given to increase red cell mass and haemoglobin levels. This may be used in combination with acute normovolaemic haemodilution where 2–3 units of blood are removed at the beginning of surgery and replaced with crystalloid/colloid. During surgery, less haemoglobin is lost per unit of blood volume lost. The blood removed prior to surgery can be retransfused at the end of surgery or once haemostasis is achieved. Peroperatively a cell salvage technique can be used, where blood recovered from suction is washed, spun and processed for transfusion back to the patient. The technique is not without risk/complications which include progressive loss of bicarbonate, electrolyte imbalance, and air embolus. Concerns exist about the use of this technique in patients undergoing surgery for cancer.

The anaesthetic technique may be modified. Surgical blood loss can be reduced by hypotensive anaesthesia. The acceptance of low haemoglobin levels (even as low as 5 g/dl in selected patients) reduces the need for transfusion.

Pharmacological adjuncts may have a role in reducing the

need for transfusion. For example prophylactic use of aprotinin and tranexamic acid to enhance coagulation. Artificial oxygen carriers such as perfluorocarbon may be used as a blood substitute. These techniques are still at a research stage at this time.

Viva hints

There are many complications of blood transfusion and these should be subdivided into categories. The above classification is only an example, other classifications could include immune/non-immune or uncommon (life threatening)/common (non-life threatening) The question may be used as a lead into many other questions such as massive blood transfusion, immunology of blood, physiology of clotting.

Q3. You are scheduled to anaesthetize for a urology list. The first patient is a 5–year-old for a circumcision. What premedication would you use?

The premedication I would give to this child would depend on the psychological state of the child when seen on the ward and the anaesthetic induction plan. I would apply EMLA cream topically over two visible veins on the dorsum of the hands or the antecubital fossa to all children of this age. If the child was nervous, upset or uncooperative on the preoperative visit I would consider a sedative or anxiolytic premedicant. I would use midazolam syrup (0.5 mg/kg). If an inhalational induction were planned, due to anticipated difficult intravenous cannulation, I would add an anticholinergic agent such as atropine (20 µg/kg orally) to the midazolam. I would advise that any other regular medication, such as antiepileptic drugs, should be taken on the morning of surgery.

Where I work the anaesthetists often use temazepam, do you have any experience of this?

The examiner may ask you questions about your anaesthetic experience. Answer truthfully, you cannot be expected to have seen every technique. Don't answer yes if you haven't experienced the situation/scenario being discussed as the question is often a leader into further questions which may catch you out.

Yes, I have used it. I generally give it at a dose of 0.5–0.75 mg/kg up to a maximum of 20 mg orally.

What are the advantages and disadvantages of using midazolam as a premedicant?

The main advantage of midazolam is that it has a rapid onset of 10–20 min and therefore is useful in situations where there may not be time for a slower onset drug such as temazepam. Such situations may include the first patient on a day care list or when unscheduled changes are made to a routine list. However, the duration of action is also relatively short and therefore timing is very important. Midazolam produces a good level of sedation in uncooperative patients for intravenous cannulation or an inhalational induction. It may be given orally or intranasally (although I have never seen it given by this route).

In the past antihistamines were used as premedicants in children, this seems to be less popular now. What are the pros and cons of antihistamines as premeds?

The use of antihistamines as a premedication relies on the sedative side effect of the drug. They are not anxiolytic like the benzodiazepines. The antihistamines have multiple effects including anticholinergic and antidopaminergic effects. These effects are useful for drying secretions and would in theory provide an antiemetic effect. The main problem of using antihistamines for their sedative action is that a moderately large dose has to be used. This may require a large volume of syrup to be given unless concentrated solutions are used. The drugs also have a prolonged duration of action and sedation may persist into the postoperative period. Hyperactivity has also been reported in some children.

Changing the subject slightly, what perioperative analgesia would you use?
Circumcisions are usually performed as day cases. I would use a 'day-case' approach to analgesia which would incorporate a short acting opioid such as fentanyl, combined with a local anaesthetic block such as a penile block. I would then use a combination of oral analgesics such as paracetamol (10–15 mg/kg – 6 hourly) and/or a non-steroidal anti-inflammatory such as ibuprofen (5 mg/kg – 6 hourly) for postoperative analgesia.

How would you perform a penile nerve block?
I would first gain consent after explaining the procedure to the accompanying parent/carer. The procedure is performed when the child is anaesthetized using a sterile technique. A standard 23 gauge Quinke needle may be used. The lower border of the pubic symphysis is palpated with the non-dominant hand and the needle is inserted in the midline at an angle of 30°. The needle is directed past the lower border of the pubic symphysis towards the base of the penis. After aspiration to exclude intravascular injection about 5 ml of 0.5% bupivacaine (*without adrenaline*) is injected to block the dorsal nerve. A further 1–2 ml of local anaesthetic may be injected around the base of the penis (like a ring block) to block the ventral nerve.

What are the complications of this block?
This question may be asked of any local anaesthetic nerve block. Complications should be classified into (1) general complications of any block such as failure, haematoma, infection, (2) specific complications of the block including damage to local structures, and (3) complications associated with the use of local anaesthetic such as intravascular injection and systemic toxicity.

The complications of this block would include general complications such as local bruising/haematoma and local infection. Systemic local anaesthetic toxicity may occur due to inadvertent intravascular injection or local absorption if the toxic dose is exceeded. If the corpora cavernosa are damaged by the needle, a large haematoma may develop.

What other local anaesthetic techniques could be used for a circumcision?
A 'caudal' may be used for this operation, alternatively EMLA cream may be applied locally around the site of surgery.

Would you use a caudal as part of a day-case anaesthetic?
A 'caudal' gives superior analgesia, however this is associated with a sensory-motor block in the lower limbs. If this block is prolonged there may be a loss of proprioception and unsteadiness on walking. This could cause a delay in discharge and even unplanned admission. Thus if a caudal is planned as part of the anaesthetic technique the patient should preferably be done in the early part of a morning list. I would counsel the parent/carer about the potential benefits of a caudal but warn them of postoperative weakness in the legs and that this occasionally leads to delay in discharge and overnight admission.

Related questions/discussion

• *Questions on premedication are common and may be clinical (as above) or may be asked in the pharmacology viva.*
• *You could be asked to expand on EMLA cream, e.g. definition, dose, constitution and side effects. Remember it contains 2.5% prilocaine which can cause methaemoglobinaemia in small babies who tend to eat dressings!*

Thank you (is it coffee time yet?).
Thank you (is the pub open yet?).

Viva Examination B

VIVA I (PHARMACOLOGY/PHYSIOLOGY)
EXAMINER I – PHARMACOLOGY

QI. Drugs acting on receptors may be classified as agonists or antagonists. Can you define these terms?

An agonist is a drug or agent which binds to a receptor producing a change in conformation resulting in a response measured as a desired therapeutic or toxic effect. Agonists can be competitive (reversible) or non-competitive.

An antagonist produces no effect when it binds to a receptor. The antagonist will compete for receptor binding sites and prevent or decrease pharmacological responses to agonists.

What is the relationship between the drug concentration and response?
A hyperbolic curve describes the relationship *(draw curve – Figure 3.6a)* where the response rapidly increases when the

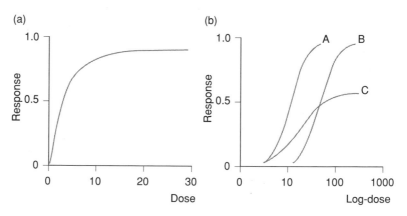

Figure 3.6 (a) Example of a dose-response curve. (b) Log-dose-response curves for (A) pure agonist, (B) agonist + competitive antagonist and (C) partial agonist.

drug is initially introduced, as unoccupied receptors are rapidly occupied. The rate of increase slows down as the number of unoccupied receptors falls until the maximum response is seen once all the receptors are occupied. At this point no further increase in response is seen, however much the concentration of drug is increased.

We usually represent this relationship by plotting the log-dose versus the response. Can you draw this curve?
If the response is plotted against the log-dose *(draw curve A – Figure 3.6b)* a sigmoid curve is obtained. This is advantageous because a linear relationship occurs for a large part of the response allowing comparison between different drugs of different potency.

Can you draw on your diagram the effect of adding a competitive antagonist?
Draw curve B – Figure 3.6b and explain...

The curve is shifted to the right, so that a higher concentration of agonist is required to produce the response. The curves are parallel indicating the competitive nature of the interaction. The maximum effect (i.e. the plateau of the curve) can be obtained if the concentration of agonist is high enough.

What does the slope of the curve tell you?
A steep slope indicates a large increase in effect for a small increase in concentration. A shallow curve indicates the drug concentration has to be increased by a large amount to produce a small effect. When different drugs have parallel curves, they have similar affinity for the receptor producing the effect.

What does the maximum response represent?
Maximal receptor occupancy occurs at this point. The measured effect is a reflection of the efficacy of the drug. No fur-

ther increase in response can be produced by increasing the concentration of agonist.

Which point on the curve would you use to compare the effect of different agonists?
Any point may be used but it is logical to use the linear part of the curve and traditionally the 50% response (P_{50}) is used. This comparison describes the potency of the drugs being compared.

What is a partial agonist?
A partial agonist is a drug which binds to a receptor to produce a response. However the response is less than the maximum possible (with a full agonist) regardless of the concentration of drug. The curves are not parallel indicating different affinities for the receptor. *(You should offer to draw this on your graph; curve C – Figure 3.6b.)*

What is a physiological antagonist?
This is a drug/agent which exerts its effect by physiological mechanisms. For example neostigmine acts by inhibiting acetylcholinesterase. The resultant rise in ACh antagonizes /reverses the neuromuscular block produced by non-depolarizing muscle relaxants.

All the discussion so far has involved drug/receptor interactions, by what other mechanisms do drugs exert their action?
You should list these and give an example of each.

Drugs act by the following means:

- Chemical reaction, e.g. antacids to neutralize gastric acid
- Enzyme inhibition to reduce production of endogenous products, e.g. ACE inhibitors which inhibit angiotensin-converting enzyme used in the treatment of hypertension
- Osmotic effect to expand plasma volumes or to promote diuresis, e.g. mannitol
- Adsorption, where a drug acts as a binding agent to prevent

toxic effects, e.g. activated charcoal used in some types of drug overdose
- Disruption of cell function, e.g. antibiotics which may disrupt cell wall/membrane function or chemotherapeutic treatments in malignancy which disrupt nucleic acid synthesis

Q2. What pharmacological methods are available for producing hypotension during anaesthesia?

It is very important to classify this question as there are many different groups of drugs involved.

I would divide these up into drugs with specific hypotensive action and drugs which produce hypotension as a secondary action.
Drugs with specific hypotensive action include:

- Vasodilators acting on the endothelial wall, e.g. nitrates, nitroprusside and hydrallazine
- β-blockers, e.g. esmolol
- α-blockers, e.g. phentolamine
- Calcium channel antagonists, e.g. amlodipine and nimodipine

Drugs which produce hypotension as a secondary action or side effect include:

- Volatile anaesthetic agents
- Neuromuscular antagonists with ganglion blocking or histamine releasing properties
- Neuroleptic drugs with alpha-blocking effects

Discuss the pharmacodynamic actions of the drugs acting on the endothelial wall?
Drugs acting on the endothelial wall exert their effect by increasing nitric oxide which was previously labelled endothelial dependent relaxing factor (EDRF). This reacts with thiols in the muscle cell to produce nitrothiols which stimulate the production of cyclic guanosine monophosphate (cGMP) from

guanosine triphosphate (GTP). cGMP is an intracellular messenger resulting in endothelial smooth muscle relaxation and vasodilatation.

How do β–blockers produce hypotension?

β-blockers have negative inotropic and chronotropic effects on the heart. They produce hypotension since:

$$BP = CO \times TPR \text{ and } CO = HR \times SV$$

where BP = blood pressure, CO = cardiac output, TPR = total peripheral resistance and SV = stroke volume.

β-blockers reduce both heart rate and contractility (stroke volume), thus producing hypotension by reductions in cardiac output.

Which drugs are commonly used as hypotensives in anaesthetic practice?

All the volatile agents currently available produce an element of hypotension and anaesthetists commonly use this property to induce hypotension. The hypotension produced by these drugs is secondary to central inhibition of the vasomotor centre, direct peripheral vasodilatation and negative inotropic effects on the heart.

Nitrates such as glyceryl trinitrate are predominantly venodilators but produce arteriolar dilatation at higher concentrations. They are given by infusion (50 mg in 50 ml) at a rate of 1–10 mg/h titrated to effect.

Hydrallazine is commonly used in anaesthetic practice, particularly in obstetric anaesthesia. It has central and peripheral effects. The peripheral action is mediated by cGMP which accumulates in the smooth muscle resulting in relaxation. It may be given by infusion or bolus and has a relatively long duration of action.

Several β-blockers may be used to produce hypotension during anaesthesia. It is possible to use propranolol, but this has a relatively long half-life and is therefore not readily titratable. It has a high oral first-pass metabolism and so the intravenous dose is much smaller (about 1 mg). Labetalol is commonly used and has the additional advantage of having some α-blocking effects; it is given by bolus (5–10 mg) or infusion (10–150 mg/h). Esmolol is a β-blocker with an ultrashort half-life of about 7 min; its effect is readily titrated.

Occasionally it may be necessary to use nitroprusside. It causes vasodilatation by increasing nitric oxide. It is a difficult drug to use as it is broken down by light, and there is a serious risk of cyanide toxicity with cumulative doses.

(Don't dig yourself into a hole with nitroprusside, it is rarely used nowadays and if you are not confident leave it to the end of your answer and hopefully the examiner will not ask you any detailed questions on its use.)

You mentioned that esmolol has a very short half-life. How is this achieved?
Esmolol is a β-blocker which contains an ester bond. It is rapidly hydrolysed by red cell esterase to inactive metabolites.

Do you know any other drugs with similar properties?
Remifentanil is an ultrashort acting opioid metabolized by tissue and plasma esterases to inactive metabolites which are excreted in the urine. Suxamethonium consists of two acetylcholine molecules bound by an ester linkage. It too is rapidly hydrolysed by plasma cholinesterase and has a short half-life of 3–5 min.

Viva hints

Listen to questions about hypotension closely and answer the question asked. For example, the above question arises in the pharmacology viva and greater emphasis should be placed on the pharmacology of the drugs used. The question could come up in the clinical viva where a more holistic approach is required of which pharmacology plays only a small part of the overall achievement of hypotension. Such an answer could be structured as follows:

* *Preoperatively: Anxiolytic premed to decrease circulating catecholamines. Avoid premedication causing a tachycardia.*

- *Induction: Should be 'smooth', therefore adequate induction dose, avoid coughing at intubation, attenuate stress response to laryngoscopy, e.g. opioid, local anaesthetic, β-blocker.*
- *Maintenance: Position – venous drainage. Hypotension by anaesthetic agent, regional techniques, pharmacological adjuncts.*
- *Postoperatively: attenuate stress response to extubation, adequate analgesia.*

Q3. Discuss the routes by which opioid analgesia may be given.

There are a large number of different routes. In this situation it is reasonable to start with the most common progressing to more complex methods and end with one or two novel routes if time allows. Include a brief discussion about the advantages and disadvantages of each.

Opioids are given enterally or parenterally. The enteral route is commonly used for chronic pain situations where absorption is predictable. In the acute situation absorption is unpredictable due to delayed gastric emptying and this route is rarely used for postoperative pain.

Yes that's right. Talk about the parenteral routes.
The intramuscular route is commonly used for postoperative analgesia. There is vast experience with this mode of administration and it is relatively safe from the point of view of potential complications. However, intermittent intramuscular opioid administration when the patient requests analgesia is far from ideal. It is difficult to titrate the dose according to the patient's needs. Further, delays may occur with drug administration and the pharmacokinetics of this method result in peaks and troughs in plasma opioid levels leading to inconsistent pain control.

Opioids may be given by the intravenous route. For example bolus intravenous opioid injections are commonly used in the postoperative recovery area to achieve rapid control of pain. Continuous intravenous opioid infusions achieve stable

plasma opioid levels but require a high level of supervision and clinical observation in high dependency areas or the intensive care unit. Intravenous opioids may be administered by 'patient controlled analgesia'. *(Look or wait for prompts from the examiner as to whether they want you to expand at this point, otherwise continue with other routes.)*
Opioids may be given by subcutaneous infusion. However, absorption may be variable due to changes in skin blood flow which is reduced in patients with high levels of circulating catecholamines that occurs secondary to pain or blood loss. In this situation a large drug 'reservoir' may build up which will be absorbed when skin perfusion is restored leading to the potential for opioid overdose.
Opioids can be given into the epidural and intrathecal space. Due to the complex nature of administration together with the possibility of potentially life threatening complications, this practice is confined to complex surgical procedures. Ideally the patient is nursed in a high dependency area, if this is not available strict protocols combined with intense nurse training to recognize early complications are required.
Novel routes of opioid administration are currently undergoing research to evaluate their potential uses including intranasal diamorphine, transdermal fentanyl patches and iontophoretic transdermal transfer *(where transdermal passage of drug is enhanced by an electrical current)* of morphine and fentanyl.

List the side effects of opioid administration

Listen to the question, which has asked for a list. You should be able to give a concise answer to this straightforward question. If you ramble too much you will lose valuable time for scoring marks in other parts of the viva.

The side effects of morphine include respiratory depression, nausea and vomiting, sedation, constipation, itching, urinary retention, and miosis.

What methods are available for monitoring respiratory depres-

sion in a patient receiving an epidural infusion of opioid and local anaesthetic?
The majority of methods commonly used are imperfect as significant respiratory impairment, i.e. reduced minute volume with CO_2 retention may be present before the respiratory rate drops. 'Routine' hourly respiratory rate monitoring may miss sudden changes in respiratory rate.

The respiratory rate may be continuously monitored by changes in the chest impedance measured by the ECG electrodes.

Arterial or expired CO_2 monitoring is probably the gold standard, but is difficult in a ward setting in spontaneously breathing patients.

Sedation scores are useful as sedation usually proceeds significant respiratory depression and is therefore more sensitive than respiratory rate monitoring.

Remember pulse oximetry is of little value for detecting respiratory depression, particularly if the patient is breathing supplementary oxygen.

Discuss the pharmacokinetics of a bolus dose of morphine administered into the epidural space.
The epidural space contains a large element of adipose tissue and is highly vascular due to a large plexus of epidural veins. The initial spread of the drug within the epidural space will depend on the initial volume in which the drug is diluted. Once in the space the morphine will diffuse into three compartments: (1) the epidural veins, (2) the epidural adipose tissue, and (3) through the dura into the CSF and then into neural tissue within the spinal canal. The rate and degree at which these movements occur are determined by the relative water and lipid solubility of the opioid. In the case of morphine, which has a relatively high water solubility and low lipid affinity, limited amounts of drug will diffuse into the epidural fat space. Diffusion into the epidural veins will be high and peak plasma concentrations are seen at 15–30 min. Diffusion through the dura is relatively slow compared to other opioids

but once this occurs the water-soluble morphine tends to remain in this compartment. From here it can diffuse within the CSF in a cephalad direction. Potentially high levels of morphine can reach the brain stem causing profound respiratory depression. This process takes many hours and this late respiratory depression can occur from 12–24 h after epidural administration.

How do opioids administered into the epidural space exert an analgesic action?
Epidural opioids exert their action by interaction with opioid receptors. These are located in the spinal cord and brain. The interaction with opioid receptors in the spinal cord is due to local diffusion from the epidural space. There is also some interaction with supratentorial opioid receptors in the brain from epidural opioid which is absorbed into the systemic circulation via the epidural veins.

Related questions

- *Discuss the structure/function of opioid receptors.*
- *Discuss the classification and distribution of opioid receptors.*
- *Discuss the use of patient controlled analgesia, advantages, disadvantages and side-effects.*
- *Discuss other drugs which may be administered in the epidural space.*

EXAMINER 2 – PHYSIOLOGY

Q1. Imagine that you have just accidentally spilt some boiling water on the back of your hand. Explain the nerve pathways which are involved in the sensation of pain.

Remember that pain is a conscious experience. All pre-cortical nerve transmission should be referred to as nociception.

The boiling water will stimulate peripheral nociceptors in the skin. Activation of these results in generation of nerve action potentials in nociceptive afferent nerve fibres. There are two types of afferent nociceptive nerve fibre. Aδ fibres are thinly myelinated and have a faster conduction velocity than the unmyelinated C fibres which form the other group of fibre. The action potential travels along the afferent neurone, whose cell body is in the dorsal root ganglion, to the dorsal horn of the spinal cord. These first-order neurones synapse in the dorsal horn and the action potential continues in the second-order nociceptive neurones. The second-order neurones cross in the spinal cord to the contra-lateral side and travel up the spinal cord in the spinothalamic tract. These second-order neurones synapse in the thalamus and the action potential continues in third-order nociceptive neurones. These radiate in the thalamo-cortical radiation to the cortex. Once the impulse arrives in the cortex the sensation of pain is felt.

What is the structure of the peripheral nociceptor?
Nociceptors have no specific structure – they are bare nerve endings which are found in most tissues throughout the body.

How does the boiling water trigger a nerve action potential?
When the boiling water contacts the skin there will be local cellular damage due to the thermal energy. Intracellular contents such as ATP and K^+ are released which depolarize the cell membrane of the bare nerve ending. Once the threshold is reached, a nerve action potential is triggered. Additionally the cell damage triggers a local inflammatory response with release of inflammatory mediators such as serotonin, bradykinin and histamine. These interact with nerve cell membrane ion channel proteins, changing the permeability so that the resting membrane potential is nearer the threshold for action potential generation. The nociceptor is sensitized, making it more likely that potentials will be generated at increased frequency.

When you burn yourself there is often a sharp pain followed by a prolonged burning sensation after. Can you explain the physiological basis of these different sensations?
The initial sharp pain, often labelled 'fast pain', is thought to be transmitted by the myelinated Aδ fibres. These synapse

with second-order nociceptive afferents and also with motor fibres to form a protective reflex synapse loop resulting in withdrawal from the painful stimulus. The burning pain after is thought to result from transmission of nociceptive impulses in the unmyelinated C-fibres which have a slow conduction velocity. This prolonged burning pain is maintained by the local inflammatory response which sensitizes the nerve endings. This has a protective function in that the damaged tissue is immobilized and protected so no further damage occurs.

You have suggested that after a burn (or a scar from surgery) the peripheral nociceptors become more sensitive. What other changes occur in the nociceptive system?

This question is asking about 'wind-up' and 'plasticity', you will need to mention these key words.

The nociceptive system is not a 'fixed-wire' system and can adapt according to the severity and duration of the nociceptive stimulus. This phenomenon is called plasticity. The system can adapt to become more sensitive so that it is more likely that nociceptive action potentials will be generated. When they are generated by a stimulus they discharge at a higher frequency. This is labelled 'wind-up'. The peripheral nociceptors are sensitized by local inflammation *(you have already discussed this so don't repeat yourself)*. Wind-up also occurs at the level of the dorsal horn. Repeated afferent nociceptive input results in the release of 'slow' neurotransmitters at the synapse. These sensitize the second-order neurone synaptic membrane by generating slow excitatory membrane potentials which raise the membrane resting potential towards the action potential threshold. They also mediate change by second messenger systems such as cyclic AMP and calcium. The increased sensitivity of the second-order neurone may cause normally non-painful stimuli (such as light touch) whose afferent neurones synapse in the vicinity to trigger nociceptive action potentials in the second-order neurone – this is called allodynia. Additionally painful stimuli from nociceptive afferents will be enhanced – hyperalgesia.

What inhibitory factors play a part at the dorsal horn?
Inhibitory receptors are located on the pre- and post-synaptic membranes at the synapse between first- and second-order neurones.
Opioid receptors are located on pre- and post-synaptic membranes. Stimulation of these results in opening of K^+ channels via a G-protein link. Potassium efflux results in hyperpolarization of the post-synaptic membrane and inhibition of nociceptive transmission. Additionally, opioid-induced closure of calcium channels reduces calcium influx at the nerve terminal which inhibits neurotransmitter release.
GABA receptors are located on the pre- and post-synaptic membranes. Stimulation of these open ligand-gated chloride channels. Chloride influx into the cell (increased negative ions) causes hyperpolarization.
α_2 adrenoceptors are located on the post-synaptic membrane and act via an inhibitory transmembrane G-protein linked to potassium ion channels, and potassium efflux causes hyperpolarization.
Descending inhibitory neurones also influence nociceptive transmission at the dorsal horn. They arise supratentorially in the peri-aqueductal grey matter.

Q2. Describe the factors that affect the distribution of water/fluids across a capillary membrane.

The capillary wall is composed of endothelial cells, which have tight intercellular junctions. The membrane is freely soluble to water, certain ions and small molecules less than 8 nm in diameter. The distribution of water across the membrane is dependent on the balance of hydrostatic and osmotic forces across the membrane. These were originally described by Starling.

Would you like to expand on this a little more?
To explain the balance of forces across the membrane I will discuss factors which lead to fluids moving out of the capillary and those tending to keep fluids in. As the endothelial mem-

brane is freely permeable to ions the concentration of these will be similar on both sides of the capillary wall and will have little effect on fluid movements. Fluids move out of the capillary due to the hydrostatic pressure within the capillary (P_C) and the colloid osmotic pressure (π_{IC}) in the interstitial fluid. Factors keeping fluid within the capillary include the plasma osmotic pressure (π_C) and the hydrostatic pressure of the interstitial space (P_{IC}).

Can you give a value for the capillary hydrostatic pressure?
The capillary hydrostatic pressure ranges from 12 to 30 mmHg and is highest at the arteriolar side and lowest at the venous side of the capillary circulation.

What is the value of the capillary osmotic pressure and what components are responsible for this?
The capillary osmotic pressure is approximately 25 mmHg and is secondary to the plasma proteins of which albumin is the most important.

Can you bring this all together and give me an equation to summarize the overall pressure gradient across the capillary wall?
Yes, this is the difference between outward and inward pressures. The outward pressure = $P_C + \pi_{IC}$ and the inward pressure = $P_{IC} + \pi_C$ and so:

$$\text{Pressure gradient} = (P_C + \pi_{IC}) - (P_{IC} + \pi_C)$$

How is this related to the filtration rate?
The filtration rate is proportional to the pressure gradient and the filtration coefficient (K).
Thus, the filtration rate = $K \times [(P_C + \pi_{IC}) - (P_{IC} + \pi_C)]$.

Generally the amount of fluid filtered out of the capillary exceeds that reabsorbed, what happens to this fluid?
The excess fluid filtered out of the capillary is absorbed into the lymphatic system and is eventually returned to the circulation via the thoracic duct.

What other functions does the lymph system have?
In addition to returning the excess fluid filtered from the capillaries back to the circulation, it also returns protein which may leak out of the capillaries. Lymph has a protein content of 20 g/l. The lymph is also responsible for the absorption of protein and fat derived from metabolism and the GI tract. The lymphatic system has an important immune function and 'mops' up other large molecular weight molecules and foreign proteins which accumulate in inflamed tissues.

Often patients that we see preoperatively have tissue oedema. Bearing in mind the factors we have discussed, what are the potential causes and mechanisms of this?
Dependent oedema is commonly seen in the elderly. It is caused by increased capillary hydrostatic pressure which is secondary to a rise in the pressure at the venous end of the capillary circulation caused by gravity and immobility. This may be exacerbated by poor right ventricular function which causes venous congestion due to 'pump failure'.

Peripheral oedema may be secondary to volume overload when large volumes of isotonic crystalloid are given. There will be a dilution of plasma protein and a reduction in the plasma oncotic pressure.

The oedema may be secondary to hypoalbuminaemia causing a reduction in plasma oncotic pressure allowing fluid to leak out from the capillaries. Hypoalbuminaemia may be due to failure of production (e.g. liver disease) or excess loss (e.g. glomerulonephritis).

Oedema may be secondary to impaired lymph drainage. This often occurs when lymph tissue is infiltrated by tumour. This type of oedema (lymphoedema) may be regional according to the lymph channels affected.

Related questions
- *Discuss the distribution of capillary fluids in sepsis.*

- *Describe the distribution of fluid following crystalloid or colloid administration.*
- *Define and explain the differences between osmotic and oncotic pressure.*

Q3. Brain function is dependent on a constant blood flow and supply of oxygen. What is cerebral blood flow?

This is a factual question and you will be unlucky if you can't remember the figure because it will get you off to a bad start to the question. It is a basic fact that you should know. If you don't know make an educated guess or quote it as a proportion of cardiac output.

The mean cerebral blood flow (CBF) is around 50 ml/100 g/min, which is approximately 15% of the cardiac output.

How would you measure cerebral blood flow?
An application of the Fick principle may be used to estimate cerebral blood flow. This relies on the following relationship:

$$\text{Blood flow to an organ} = \frac{\text{Rate of uptake/excretion of substance}}{\text{Arterial} - \text{venous concentration difference of substance}}$$

Nitrous oxide is used as it achieves rapid equilibration within 10 min and has a blood/brain partition coefficient of approximately 1. The subject breathes a low concentration of N_2O (e.g. 10%) for 10 min. Since the partition coefficient is 1, the N_2O transferred to 100 g of brain tissue per minute (Q) is the same as the content of N_2O in 100 g of jugular venous blood. The A-V difference (D) is determined by measurement of arterial and venous samples during equilibrium. Cerebral blood flow is then calculated from Q/D.

Cerebral blood flow may also be determined by PET scanning using labelled de-oxyglucose or by flow Doppler techniques.

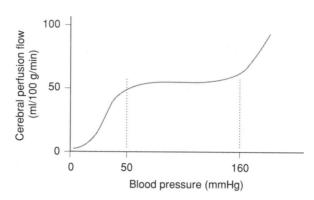

Figure 3.7 Relationship between cerebral blood flow and mean arterial pressure demonstrating autoregulation.

How is total cerebral blood flow regulated?

Total cerebral blood flow is regulated by autoregulation. This ensures that cerebral blood flow is maintained over a large range of mean blood pressures. (*You should offer to draw the graph – see Figure 3.7 and describe it as you draw it.*) This graph shows cerebral blood flow measured in ml/100 g/min on the *y*-axis and mean arterial blood pressure in mmHg along the *x*-axis. A cerebral blood flow around 50 ml/100 g/min is maintained over a pressure range of 50–150 mmHg.

Regional cerebral blood flow varies according to local brain activity and generation of metabolic by-products.

What other factors influence cerebral blood flow?

Cerebral perfusion will be reduced by raised intracranial pressure since:

Cerebral perfusion pressure = Mean arterial pressure – (venous pressure + intracranial pressure)

There is a direct relationship between arterial CO_2 and cerebral blood flow. A high $PaCO_2$ causes cerebral vasodilatation thus increasing cerebral blood flow, whilst a low $PaCO_2$ causes vasoconstriction and a reduction in cerebral blood flow.

Severe hypoxaemia causes cerebral vasodilatation which is a

last resort protective mechanism to maintain cerebral oxygen delivery in situations of extreme hypoxic stress. Arterial O_2 tension has little effect on cerebral blood flow in normal physiological circumstances.

Acidosis causes cerebral vasodilatation, a mechanism which is important in the local regulation of cerebral blood flow.

Metabolites such as adenosine and potassium result in local cerebral vasodilatation. These products of metabolism result in increased local blood flow to increase oxygen delivery in areas where it is needed.

Related questions

Special circulation questions are common in the physiology viva. You should be able to discuss the distribution of coronary and renal blood flows, and have knowledge of the fetal circulation and the changes that occur with birth.

Thank you.
Thank you.

VIVA 2 (CLINICAL MEASUREMENT, PHYSICS AND CLINICAL)

EXAMINER I – CLINICAL MEASUREMENT/PHYSICS

Q1. Outline the methods by which oxygen is stored for medical use in hospitals.

In most hospitals, oxygen is stored in liquid form and transferred to the hospital via a network of pipelines. Oxygen is also stored as a gas in cylinders. These are arranged in banks of cylinders to supply theatres or can be directly attached to the yolk of the anaesthetic machine.

What safety features ensure the correct delivery of oxygen to the anaesthetic machine?

Divide this into pipeline gases and cylinders.

Only certified engineers are allowed to work on medical gas pipelines and pharmacy has responsibilities for checking the purity of pipeline oxygen. The pipelines between the wall outlet and the anaesthetic machine are colour coded (white for oxygen) and reinforced so they cannot be occluded. At the wall outlet, Schroder valves are designed so that the outlet will only accept the probe appropriate for the gas pipeline for which it is intended. At the machine end, the pipeline is attached via a gas-specific non-interchangeable screw thread (NIST) which is a 'permanent' connection which can only be released with special tools.

Oxygen cylinders are colour coded (black with white shoulders) and are labelled on the cylinder valve block and on the cylinder itself. The valve block and cylinder yolk have a pin index system whereby pins protruding from the yolk fit into holes on the cylinder valve block. Each gas has a unique pattern/position for the two pins ensuring correct cylinder placement.

How is oxygen stored as a liquid?

To store oxygen as a liquid it has to be cooled. It is stored in a large upright flask which is similar to a vacuum flask to

prevent excessive warming of the liquid which is stored at
–187°C. As oxygen is required it evaporates from the liquid.
Thus the apparatus is called a Vacuum Insulated Evaporator
(VIE).

*If you know about critical temperature you could volunteer this
information at this stage as it would be likely that the next question will ask about it...*

**At what temperature does oxygen have to be stored to remain in
liquid form?**
It has to be below –119°C which is the critical temperature.

What is the definition of critical temperature?
The critical temperature is the temperature *above* which it is
impossible to liquefy a gas by pressure alone.

**What processes occur in the VIE when oxygen is required for the
hospital pipeline system?**
The space above the liquid oxygen is filled with oxygen vapour.
This is at a pressure of approximately 10 atm. This is generated because the VIE cannot be totally insulated and therefore
heat energy is absorbed and vaporization occurs. As oxygen is
required this gas is drawn off and replaced as further evaporation occurs.

What happens if demand outstrips the above process?
The vaporization described above may not produce enough
gaseous oxygen during high demand, in this situation the pressure in the VIE drops and results in the opening of a valve to
allow liquid oxygen into a superheater evaporator to enhance
the rate of vaporization.

How is oxygen stored in oxygen cylinders?
The cylinders are stored at room temperature, which is well
above the critical temperature for oxygen, thus it is stored in
gaseous form under high pressure (137 atm).

Is the anaesthetic machine exposed to this pressure?
No, there is a reducing valve distal to the oxygen cylinder inlet
to reduce the pressure to 400 kPa, which is also the pressure of
oxygen in the pipeline.

How does a pressure reducing or regulating valve work?
*If you can draw this, offer to do so – Figure 3.8. Explain the
principles as you draw it.*

This valve works by balancing the force of a spring against a
desired gas pressure transmitted as a force on a diaphragm. As
the pressure (at the desired reduced pressure) in the low pressure chamber falls, pressure of the spring pushes the
diaphragm. The diaphragm is connected to a smaller valve
controlling the output from a high pressure chamber so that it
is possible to achieve a low pressure.

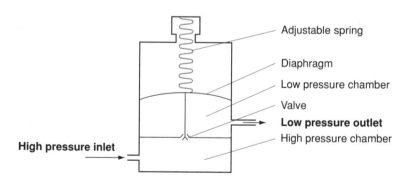

Figure 3.8 Simplified diagram of pressure regulating (pressure
reducing) valve.

Tips and allied questions

*Supply of gases is an important and popular exam question. You
could also be asked about...*

- *Construction and safety of gas cylinders*
- *Manufacture, supply and storage of nitrous oxide*
- *Entonox, supply, storage, safety + pseudo-critical temperature.*

Q2. When patients undergo prolonged surgery they often get cold. By what mechanisms do patients lose heat during surgery?

There are four main routes for heat loss.

1. Radiation is the transfer of heat energy between objects which are not touching. Infrared energy 'radiates' from the relatively warm patient to surrounding colder objects. This is the most significant mode of heat loss accounting for around 40% of total heat loss.
2. Convection is the transfer of heat energy to the air layer surrounding the patient. As this air warms, it becomes less dense and rises to be replaced by colder air and so on, resulting in net heat loss from the body. This mode of heat loss is increased if large surface areas are exposed and the air surrounding the patient is rapidly circulating, e.g. in theatres with laminar air flow systems.
3. Conduction is the transfer of heat energy between objects in contact with each other. In theatres this occurs from the patient to the operating table or the patient's blood warming cold intravenous fluids.
4. Evaporation is an important mode of heat loss. It occurs when a liquid evaporates. The energy required for molecules to leave a liquid phase to become a vapour results in transfer of energy and loss of heat. In the clinical situation, heat is lost from the evaporation of sweat and body fluids on the skin and exposed mucosal surfaces. Further heat (up to 10% of the total) is lost from the lungs where dry anaesthetic gases become saturated with water vapour (to saturated vapour pressure at body temperature).

What methods are available for measuring the patient's temperature?

This question doesn't specifically relate to theatres, therefore mention other methods used in clinical practice.

In the past, simple mercury thermometers were commonly used. These utilize the change in volume of a liquid with temperature. There are safety issues with the use of mercury, due to its toxic properties and alcohol may be substituted in its place. Alcohol is not useful for measuring high temperatures as it boils at around 78°C.

Dial thermometers work on the principle of unequal expansion of a bimetallic strip which can be calibrated to measure temperature.

A Bourdon gauge can be used to measure temperature, it relies on the expansion of mercury or a volatile agent in a sensing probe causing a change in pressure or volume which can be calibrated against change in temperature.

Electrical methods are commonly used. They utilize the following principles:

- Change in resistance since electrical resistance of a metal increases in a linear manner with increasing temperature.
- Changes in resistance that occur with temperature that take place across a thermistor.
- Changes in voltage across a thermocouple. In this method the voltage produced at the junction of two dissimilar metals varies with temperature and is compared with a reference junction held at a constant temperature to give a temperature reading.

How is the patient's temperature measured in theatre, what sites are chosen and what are the problems with each technique?

It is possible to measure the patient's peripheral temperature and/or core temperature. Often both are measured to give an indication of peripheral heat loss. This comparison will also be dependent on peripheral perfusion to some extent.

Skin temperature is usually measured by the simple application of a temperature probe to the patient's skin.

Core temperature may be measured by a probe inserted at several sites including:

- The oesophagus, where the probe should ideally be placed in the lower part of the oesophagus. At this point there is a close anatomical proximity with the aorta so there is a good indication of core blood temperature. It is difficult to know exactly where the end of the probe is situated. If it is too high it is potentially cooled by respiratory gases in the adjacent trachea giving an underestimation of core temperature.

• The nasopharynx is commonly used during anaesthesia as it is readily accessible. However it is less accurate than the oesophageal probe.

• The tympanic membrane which gives a good estimation of intracerebral temperature, provided there isn't too much wax in the ear. It is possible to obtain fast response times but there is a danger of damage to the tympanic membrane if incorrectly used.

• Intravascular probes using the thermistor in a pulmonary artery catheter will give a very good indication of core temperature. This technique has a rapid response time and is considered the gold standard, although considerable skill is required for insertion of the PA catheter and due to the invasive nature of the technique can only be used when other measurements are made necessitating the insertion of a PA catheter.

• Rectal temperature has been used, however the temperature measured can vary according to heat generated from gut blood flow and gut flora and cooling due to venous blood returning from the legs to the adjacent veins in the pelvis. The technique will also give inaccurate readings if the probe is insulated by faeces.

What methods are available for minimizing heat loss from the patient in theatres?

You can classify this question by the modes of heat loss you have described above or by active and passive techniques.

Heat loss via radiation may be minimized by covering the patient with a reflective foil 'space blanket' which reflects the heat energy radiating from the patient back to the patient. Heat may be transferred to the patient by infrared radiant heaters situated above the patient. These are commonly used in paediatric anaesthesia due to the vulnerability of neonates and small babies losing heat due to their relatively large surface area to body ratio.

Heat loss by convection may be minimized by ensuring that the air in theatres is at a reasonable temperature. A compromise has to be reached by minimizing heat loss by this route and the comfort of the theatre and surgical team. The air surrounding the patient may be actively warmed by blowing warm air through a perforated blanket placed over the patient.

Heat loss by conduction may be minimized by an active warming mattress placed under the patient. These are usually heated electrically or by circulating water. Care must be taken to ensure that the blanket doesn't over heat causing burns. Heat loss by conduction of the patient's warm blood with cold intravenous fluids can be reduced by warming intravenous fluids by passing them across a controlled temperature heating plate prior to infusion. This is particularly important when large volumes of fluid or blood stored at 4°C are given. Warming of fluids used for irrigation, e.g. during cystoscopy will also reduce heat loss from conduction.

Evaporative heat loss from open surgical sites is difficult to control. Evaporative heat loss from respiratory gases may be reduced by the use of heat moisture exchangers and by the use of the circle system which warms circulating gases due to the chemical reaction occurring in the soda lime.

Q3. What methods are available for the measurement of blood pressure?

These may be divided into direct (invasive) and indirect (non-invasive) techniques. The indirect methods may be manual or automated.

How does an automated non-invasive blood pressure (NIBP) machine work?

This machine has a single occlusive cuff with a dual sensing valve. The cuff is usually placed around the patient's upper arm over the brachial artery. The machine pumps air into the cuff to a pressure of 20–30 mmHg above the previous systolic

BP reading so that the artery is occluded by external pressure. It then deflates in a slow controlled manor through a bleed valve. As the occlusive pressure drops below the systolic BP, arterial pulsations are transmitted via the cuff to a pressure transducer. These pulsations increase in strength around the mean arterial pressure and diminish and become undetectable at the diastolic pressure, rather like Korotkov sounds heard during manual measurement.

Using an algorithm the machine calculates three pressures as follows *(see Figure 3.9)*:

- Systolic BP – appearance of pulsations
- Mean arterial BP – pressure at which pulsations have maximum amplitude
- Diastolic BP – where pulsations have declined to less than 80% of maximum.

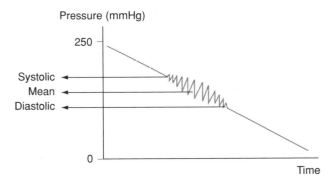

Figure 3.9 Graph of non-invasive sensed cuff pressure (pulsations exaggerated) showing determination of (A) systolic, (B) mean and (C) diastolic blood pressure.

What are the problems of using this device?
Correct estimation of BP is dependent on the correct cuff size being selected. If the cuff is too wide the pressure is underestimated and if it is too narrow the BP is overestimated. The cuff should cover two-thirds of the length of the upper arm. The correct detection of the beginning and end-points of

pulsation is dependent on a regular cardiac cycle. The device is inaccurate if the cardiac cycle is irregular, e.g. in atrial fibrillation or with multiple ventricular ectopics. The NIBP will be inaccurate at low pressures due to difficulty in identifying weak pulsations. If the BP fluctuates widely the cuff inflation pressure may be insufficient if the BP has risen significantly since the previous measurement. In this case pulsations will be present at the initial cuff inflation pressure and the cycle has to start again at a higher pressure. This leads to delay in determining an accurate pressure.

What are the indications for invasive blood pressure measurement?
Invasive blood pressure measurements are indicated in the following situations:

• To measure beat to beat variability in situations of potential cardiac instability such as during cardiac and vascular surgery
• To guide treatment when BP manipulation with inotropes or vasodilators is required
• To measure BP when NIBP measurements are impossible or inaccurate such as in obese patients.

As invasive BP measurement relies on an indwelling arterial cannula there is an added advantage that repeated arterial blood gas sampling may be taken.

What is required for direct arterial blood pressure measurement?
Arterial cannulation is required with a parallel-sided Teflon coated cannula. This is connected to a pressurized continuous flushing system to prevent the cannula from occluding with thrombus. The cannula is in communication with a pressure transducer by a continuous column of fluid inside a non-compliant connecting tube.

What problems may occur?
Arterial cannulation may be difficult, especially in situations where there is hypotension, or in diseased peripheral arteries present in some vascular patients.

Disconnection may result in significant blood loss if undetected for any length of time.

Arterial wall damage may result in intimal tears with the possibility of a false aneurysm developing.

Distal vascular insufficiency may develop due to peripheral arterial emboli such as thrombus dislodging from the end of the cannula or air bubbles introduced into the system.

Inadvertent drug administration is always a possibility, which can cause arterial spasm and distal ischaemia.

How do errors occur in the system?

Bubbles may occur in the system leading to damping of the arterial pressure waveform, in this situation the systolic BP will be underestimated and the diastolic overestimated.

Excess damping also occurs if the connecting tubing containing the column of fluid to the transducer is over compliant.

Incorrect levelling of the transducer may result in an inappropriate zero reference point. This is more relevant in low-pressure systems such as CVP measurement.

EXAMINER 2 − CLINICAL TOPICS

Q1. You are the anaesthetic SHO on-call. You are called to A&E to a 20-year-old motorcyclist who was knocked off his motorbike. On arrival he has a compound tibia and fibula fracture, blood coming from his nose, and a GCS of 5. What is your initial management?

This is an 'ABC' resuscitation situation in a patient with a severe head injury. State your priorities from the start and call for help at an early stage.

This patient is critically injured with a significant head injury and I would call for senior help at an early stage. My primary aims would be: to maintain oxygenation and ventilation and secure the airway to aid ventilation and reduce the risk of aspiration, to ensure an adequate circulation and cardiac output.

Once the initial resuscitation phase is completed a further examination of the patient is required (secondary survey) looking for associated potentially life threatening injuries.

You mentioned that you wish to secure the airway, How are you going to achieve this safely?
The concern with this patient is the possibility of an associated unstable cervical spine injury coupled with the fact that the patient may have a full stomach (particularly as trauma is associated with delayed gastric emptying). Intubating equipment should be checked and appropriate drugs drawn up in labelled syringes. In this situation a rapid sequence induction is required to secure the airway. The neck must be immobilized to prevent excessive movement during intubation. Two assistants are essential to correctly apply cricoid pressure and to maintain neck stability by in line cervical traction. The patient should be preoxygenated for a minimum of 3 min prior to the administration of an induction dose of intravenous anaesthetic followed by suxamethonium. It may be necessary to release the front part of the hard neck collar during this procedure to allow mouth opening. The patient's trachea should be intubated with an appropriate size cuffed tracheal tube and the lungs ventilated.

This patient was unconscious so why have you used an induction agent?
An induction agent is used in this situation to reduce the hypertensive response to laryngoscopy which would increase intracranial pressure (ICP). It would also prevent any potential awakening of the patient from the strong stimulus of laryngoscopy.

Suxamethonium increases intracranial pressure are you sure you would use this?

The examiners are testing your confidence in your answers. Do not be put off by this tactic. Remember the airway always takes first priority... Remember the balance of risk.

Suxamethonium does cause a small increase in intracranial pressure but has a significant advantage of producing profound muscle relaxation and optimum intubating conditions within 60–90 s. Further, in most patients it has a very short duration of action if intubation of the trachea is not possible.

How do you confirm correct placement of the tracheal tube?
Correct placement is confirmed by seeing the tube pass through the cords and observing the chest rising and falling with ventilation (although this can be misleading occasionally). It is necessary to listen for breath sounds in the peripheries of both lungs and checking for the absence of gurgling over the stomach. The gold standard of correct tube placement is the confirmation of CO_2 in expiratory air with the observation of consistent capnograph traces over a number of breaths.

What would you do if you couldn't intubate the trachea?
This will be along the lines of a failed intubation drill but you will not have the option of waking this patient up! State your priorities at the beginning of your answer.

A failed intubation drill should be employed with the main priority of maintaining oxygenation which will minimize the risks of secondary hypoxic brain damage and protecting the airway in a trauma patient with a potentially full stomach.

The help of a senior anaesthetist should be sought. Cricoid pressure should be maintained and ventilation attempted with the face mask. If ventilation is not possible then an *oral* airway should be inserted (a nasal airway would be contraindicated if there was a suspicion of basal skull fracture − *history of blood from nose*). If further attempts at intubation are attempted, hypoxia, hypo- and hypertension should be avoided as these all lead to secondary brain damage. If ventilation is not possible with a face mask and airway, one can consider inserting a LMA to enable ventilation. This does not protect the airway and cricoid pressure should be maintained if at all possible. By this stage one would hope that the suxamethonium was beginning to wear off and that spontaneous respiration would return. However the airway still requires intubation to allow ventilation (and thus control of CO_2) and to protect it from aspiration. Once spontaneous respiration has returned several options may be considered including:

- Further attempts at intubation by a more senior experienced anaesthetist using difficult intubation aids such as the McCoy laryngoscope
- Establishment of a surgical airway, i.e. tracheostomy, particularly if there were associated facial trauma
- Oral fibre-optic intubation (if personnel with the appropriate skill are available).

Assuming that the patient is stabilized in A&E you are informed that the patient requires transfer to a neurosurgical unit in another hospital. Explain briefly how you would prepare for this?

Assume from the preceding discussion that the patient is already intubated. A brief synopsis is required, discuss this under patient factors, equipment/monitoring/drugs and personnel/ambulance.

The patient must be stabilized for transfer *(expand if asked, i.e. fluid resuscitation in progress, inotropes as required, oxygenation maintained with basic modes of ventilation)* and no immediate surgery required such as an acute abdomen, e.g. ruptured spleen. The tracheal tube and intravenous lines must be firmly secured before transferring the patient to the ambulance stretcher. Blankets such as 'space-blankets' should be considered to minimize heat loss.

Full monitoring is required. Ideally the patient should be ventilated by portable ventilator to ensure adequate control of CO_2. A supply of drugs should be drawn up in labelled syringes with back up supplies available. Intravenous infusions should be given by pump. A self-inflating bag should be available in case of failure of ventilator/oxygen supply.

Escorting personnel should be adequately trained, confirm with the ambulance crew regarding defibrillation equipment, and confirm adequate oxygen availability and supply on-board. Finally don't forget the notes, X-rays and referral letter.

Q2. What standards of monitoring are recommended during anaesthesia?

State basic ground rules first which are:

The presence of an anaesthetist, of appropriate seniority and experience, at all times during surgery is of vital importance. Equipment should be available to monitor the correct function of the anaesthetic equipment and to monitor the vital signs of the patient.

Monitoring standards apply to any situation where anaesthesia is given both in and outside the hospital setting. The same standards of monitoring should be applied during transfers (inter- and intra hospital) and for local anaesthetic and sedation techniques.

The anaesthetist should have appropriate experience for the case. Accurate records should be kept and observations recorded at appropriate intervals (usually every 5 min). Before commencing anaesthesia, all monitors and equipment should be checked and alarms set and activated.

Correct function of the anaesthetic machine is monitored by inspired gas analysis to confirm correct delivery of oxygen and anaesthetic. An oxygen analyser with an audible alarm is mandatory. Delivery of anaesthetic should be confirmed by a vapour analyser when volatile anaesthesia is used and by visual checks of intravenous infusion sites in TIVA techniques. When intermittent positive ventilation is used, high and low pressure alarms should be used to detect abnormally high pressure and disconnection.

Monitoring the patient can be defined as routine (minimal standards) and advanced according to clinical needs. Routine monitoring stipulates that the following are used: At induction ECG, pulse oximeter, NIBP and capnograph (with nerve stimulator and temperature probes available). During anaesthesia the above plus vapour analyser. During recovery pulse oximetry plus NIBP are sufficient but ECG, nerve stimulator, temperature monitoring and capnography should be immediately available. Advanced monitoring techniques are dictated by clinical need and include monitoring CVP, PAP, cardiac output, direct (invasive) arterial pressure and spinal cord function (evoked responses during spinal surgery).

You mentioned that an oxygen analyser is essential. What methods are available for monitoring oxygen concentrations in the anaesthetic gas?
Paramagnetic analysers are commonly used in this situation. Oxygen has paramagnetic properties (attracted towards a magnetic field) related to single unpaired electrons in the outer shell. Gas for analysis passes through a chamber within a magnetic field. A dumbbell containing nitrogen (repelled by the magnetic field) will be displaced by oxygen in the sample gas, the degree of rotation will be related to the concentration of oxygen within the gas.

Mass spectrometry can be used to measure oxygen but is expensive and too bulky for clinical use.

How is oxygen measured in the patient in clinical practice?
State the commonest techniques first.
Oxygen can be measured using the following:

- Pulse oximetry is the commonest method of assessing oxygenation clinically. The technique involves the differential absorption of red and infrared light by oxy- and deoxyhaemoglobin.
- *In vitro* measurement of oxygen tension in arterial blood samples. Two common methods exist for this, the oxygen (Clarke) electrode and the galvanic fuel cell.
- Intravascular oxygen electrodes using a variant of the Clarke electrode.
- Intravascular techniques using optodes, which utilize the concentration dependent property of oxygen to reduce fluorescence of certain dyes.

• Transcutaneous oxygen electrodes which are used in neonatal practice and rely on the diffusion of oxygen from the capillaries in the dermis of the skin into an electrode.

In what situations does a pulse oximeter give an inaccurate reading?

The pulse oximeter is inaccurate at very low oxygen saturations and situations when peripheral circulation is compromised. It is prone to motion artefacts. Certain dyes (e.g. methylene blue) and pigments (such as bilirubin) may interfere with light absorption. Abnormal haemoglobin such as carboxyhaemoglobin which is pigmented red but carries little oxygen may give a relatively normal saturation reading in a situation when the blood is carrying little oxygen.

Q3. Shortly after induction of anaesthesia, the automated BP fails to record a BP. Checking the pulse reveals a barely palpable pulse. What is your initial diagnosis?

The most common cause of hypotension at induction is the negatively inotropic and vasodilatory effects of the induction agent. This may be exaggerated in patients with hypovolaemia/dehydration. Having said this, it is always important to check your anaesthetic system is delivering an adequate concentration of oxygen. A rarer but potentially life-threatening cause would be anaphylaxis.

The patient has also developed a rash so your working diagnosis is anaphylaxis. What is your initial management?

As in the previous critical incident, state your priorities at the beginning of the answer so that the examiner knows you are focused and have confidence in your management plan.

The priority of initial treatment is to maintain oxygenation and restore circulation (ABC). Senior help should be sought from the outset. The airway should be secured by tracheal intubation, particularly if there is bronchospasm which may make ventilation difficult, and the patient's lungs ventilated with 100% oxygen. If the patient has no cardiac output CPR should commence without delay. The patient should be tilted head down to encourage venous return to the heart and a rapid intravenous infusion should be established for volume replacement with crystalloid. The first line drug of choice is epinephrine (adrenaline) given as 250–500 μg boluses (2.5–5 ml of 1:10 000) until there is return of pulse.

What pharmacodynamic factors make epinephrine the first line drug of choice?
Epinephrine has mixed α- and β-adrenoceptor action. The α_1 effects include peripheral vasoconstriction which will increase the systemic vascular resistance (SVR) to restore BP. The β_1 effects will have a positive inotropic and chronotropic effect on the heart to promote cardiac output. The β_2 effects will promote bronchodilation which is particularly desirable as bronchospasm commonly occurs in anaphylaxis.

After epinephrine, what is you further management?
Second line treatment includes:

• Salbutamol for bronchospasm, which may be given as a nebulized solution or via an intravenous infusion
• Hydrocortisone (100–200 mg) is usually given for its delayed anti-inflammatory actions
• Antihistamines such as prochlorperazine are also given by intravenous bolus

Once stabilized the patient should be transferred to ITU for further supportive management depending on the course the anaphylaxis takes.

How would you confirm the diagnosis of anaphylaxis?
The initial diagnosis is by clinical signs including rapid onset of hypotension and bronchospasm accompanied by a rash.
     Once the patient is stabilized blood should be taken for analysis of mast cell tryptase, which rises in the first few min-

utes and remains raised for several hours. This will establish whether the reaction is anaphylactic. Skin tests are performed at 6–8 weeks to confirm which drug the patient is allergic to.

Once the drug causing anaphylaxis is established this should be clearly documented in the notes and the patient given a letter and advised to wear a medic alert bracelet.

Tips/hints

In many of the clinical emergency questions there will be a possibility that the factors presented in the scenario itself or the progression of the scenario would result in a cardiac arrest. The possibility should be mentioned at the outset with a brief summary of the initial management, namely institution of basic life support (Airway, Breathing, Circulation) followed by advance life support in the form of defibrillation if indicated and/or pharmacological management of arrhythmias.

Thank you (and see you in 6 months).
Thank you (I hope I never meet them again!).

4 The Objectively Structured Clinical Examinations (OSCEs)

The OSCEs test required anaesthetic skills which cannot be adequately assessed in the MCQs or in the vivas. This component of the examination consists of a series of 16 stations, each of 5 min duration, around which the candidates rotate. Currently these are divided into two batches of eight stations with a rest period at the half-way mark. Candidates also spend about 1 min at a preparation area before each station. This preparation area is a small booth with written information about the imminent station.

The stations themselves may have anatomical models, actors, photographs, pieces of equipment or other props. The candidate may be invited to describe anatomy, demonstrate a procedure or nerve block, talk to and examine patients, check equipment or simply answer a series of questions. Most, but not all, of the stations are manned by one (occasionally two) examiners who, as in the vivas, have a list of required points that the candidates have to cover. The unmanned stations (e.g. electrocardiogram or chest X-ray interpretation stations) consist of a standardized questionnaire that must be answered. A feature of the OSCEs is the presence of actors who add realism to the proceedings. They are prepared beforehand on how to behave and what role to adopt. The performance of the actors is generally stunning in its realism.

The areas tested include:

- Resuscitation
- Technical skills
- Anatomy and regional techniques
- History-taking
- Physical examination
- Communication skills

- Interpretation of results and investigations (electrocardiograms and X-rays)
- Statistics
- Anaesthetic, monitoring equipment
- Measurement devices
- Anaesthetic hazards

MARKING

Each station is marked according to the list of required points in the examiner's checklist and is thus standardized. Most stations have only one examiner present instead of the two per viva. The system is fair, however, because all the candidates on a particular day encounter the same examiner at a specific station. Each station receives a total mark out of 20 depending on its nature, with a minimum number, normally 13, required to pass the station as a whole. You have to pass 13 out of the 16 stations to pass the OSCEs completely. Some required answers or actions receive two marks if they are covered completely, with just one mark if only some aspects are covered. For example, listening to the heart might require auscultation at rest and in inspiration/expiration in order to receive both marks. The ability to score marks independently for different parts of same station means that a candidate who makes a serious error at the beginning can still redeem him/herself later on. There are often instructions to the examiner at the top of the marking sheet, e.g. what to tell the candidate or what emphasis is especially required. The number of stations passed out of the 16 stations is converted to a final score using our familiar friend of 0 = veto, 1 = poor fail, 1+ = fail, 2 = pass and 2+ = outstanding.

Technique

It is most important to remember that the majority of stations deal with routine aspects of safe clinical practice. This means the candidates are being examined about components of their practice that are given *every day* to all patients. For example, one of the stations is about checking the anaesthetic machine and its safety features. Apparently 50% of candidates fail this OSCE station. This is surprising. At every operating list that a trainee attends the anaesthetic machine should be checked according to the Association of Anaesthetists' Guidelines. If a candidate regularly checks the machine as part of normal practice this station is easy (he/she is a safe anaesthetist). If this is not done routinely and is a last minute memory exercise this station becomes a struggle.

Similarly, talking to patients and a basic clinical examination are absolutely routine. Do these properly in clinical practice every day and these stations should be absolutely straightforward.

Candidates often wonder why they should know anatomy such as that of the skull. If one manages major trauma an understanding of the origin of cerebrospinal fluid rhinorrhoea is needed. Also, knowledge of the anatomy of the orbit is

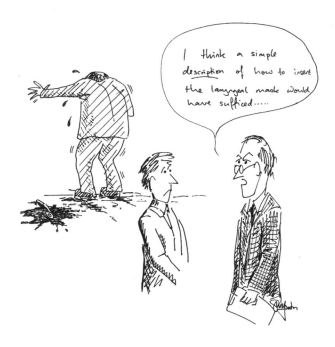

necessary if an anaesthetist is to perform local anaesthetic blocks on the eye. Basically, safe clinical practice and knowledge will lead to a pass.

What does happen, though, is the reality of 'examination nerves' and these often let a candidate down. Being mute in a communication station makes passing difficult. What can we say? We have all experienced the 'tongue stuck to the top of the dry mouth' situation but nerves can and must be overcome in the OSCEs. This is best done by practising them.

Look and behave professionally. In the 1 minute you spend at the preparation area, before meeting the examiner, read the instructions carefully and anticipate the thrust of the questions. Taking a history means taking a history and not examining the patient and examining the patient means just that. Don't forget to be polite to the 'patients.' Shake their hands, introduce yourself and talk directly to them.

We have compiled two practice OSCEs for you and have included answers with relevant marks out of 20 in parentheses. You need 13 marks out of 20 to pass each station. You can easily assess how you are performing from these mock questions. Italics have been used to give advice, when mentioning similar topic questions, or when another person is speaking in the question.

OSCE Examination A

1. COMMUNICATION SKILLS STATION

This involves discussing relevant points of management with patients in a polite and logical manner. The candidate must be able to answer questions asked by the patient using lay terms. Topics can be about any aspect of care, such as postoperative analgesia, the complications of anaesthesia or blood transfusion. Do not examine the patient - just talk at this station.

Discuss the methods of postoperative analgesia available to this 50-year-old lady who is about to undergo an elective total abdominal hysterectomy.

Introduce yourself, identify the patient, confirm the operation and check the consent. Good morning. My name is Dr .... You are scheduled to have a hysterectomy. Is that correct? (1) *Yes.* You wish to talk about postoperative pain relief for your operation? *Please.*

Your postoperative pain can and will be kept to a minimum after this operation. The operation is performed through a scar in the lower abdomen which can cause pain for several days afterwards (1).

I would like to explain the methods used to treat this. We can then decide which method will be best for you (1).

During the operation I can give you a strong pain killer, like morphine, with your anaesthetic. This drug can be continued after the operation and can be given in various forms. It used to be given via intermittent injections into the muscle of the buttock but now we commonly give it into a vein (1). This stops the pain of the injections and gives better and more continuous pain relief (1). *Good. I hate injections.*

We commonly give this via a pump which you operate and it is called a PCA pump. It allows you to give yourself painkillers when you need them. When you press the button on the pump, morphine is released and you should feel the benefit within a few minutes. The pump is set so that you cannot overdose on it (2).

Some patients are not keen on these devices as they can
make them feel quite sleepy. Morphine can cause nausea,
vomiting and constipation in susceptible patients (1).
In addition, we can supplement the pain relief with less
powerful pain killers such as paracetamol or aspirin (1).
Various formulations of these drugs exist and we can give
them either via a suppository or orally. Have your ever
taken these before? *Yes.* Did you have any side effects?
Would you have any objection to receiving a suppository?
(2) *No.*

We can also lessen the usage of these drugs by giving local
anaesthetic drugs either around the scar of the operation or
by means of epidural analgesia (2). You may have had an
epidural for the birth of your children. Do you know about
epidurals? *Yes. I did actually. It didn't work well though.* It
involves an injection into the lower back and a fine plastic
tube is inserted into the epidural space. This is a space which
surrounds the spinal cord. Epidurals provide good pain relief
and you will be pain free when you wake up. Your legs will
feel tingly and heavy for some hours afterwards (2). *Would it
be put in with me awake or asleep?* I prefer for you to be
awake as it is safer this way. There is a small risk from an
epidural of getting a severe headache as a side effect. This
can be well treated and is rare but it will slow your recovery
down (2).

We can continue with the epidural afterwards to alleviate
your pain. Mostly we do not need this form of pain relief
after this operation and normally I use a combination of
suppositories and morphine to provide adequate pain
control (1).

I hope this explains the options available. Do you have any
questions? (1) *No. As none is forthcoming you should suggest a
reasonable course of postoperative analgesia.*

So, on balance, for someone such as you, I would favour
using morphine via a PCA pump in a combination with suppositories. I shall ensure that you awaken comfortably by
administering similar drugs during the operation (1).

Further questions which may be asked by the patient could include the following:

How can you stop my sickness? I don't want an epidural – they damage your back and can paralyse you! How long will the operation hurt afterwards? How long can I have the PCA machine?

2. ECG INVESTIGATION STATION

You must be able to confidently read and interpret an ECG. Some are easy such as atrial fibrillation (what causes atrial fibrillation?) and myocardial infarction. Some, however, are more difficult! The treatment of ECG abnormalities can be asked in this section.

Look at this electrocardiogram and answer the following questions.

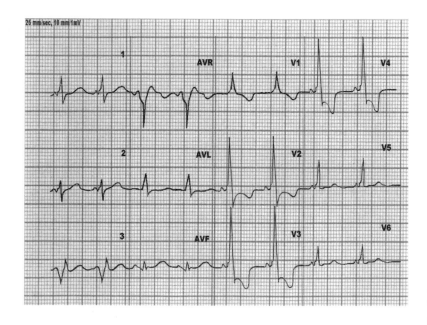

What are the characteristic findings in this ECG? (2)
A short PR (0.8 ms) interval, slurred R wave with a δ wave, an R wave in V1 and an inverted T wave in V1–4.

What is the normal PR interval? (2)
Less than 0.2 s.

What is the normal QRS complex interval? (2)
50–120 ms.

What rate is this ECG? (2)
100/min.

What is the time duration of one little square on a normal ECG? (2)
0.04 s.

What is the height of a normal QRS complex? (2)
At least 5 mm (0.5 mV) in any lead and not higher than 15.0 mm (1.5 mV) in any lead.

What is the axis of a normal ECG? (2)
−30° to +90°.

What is the axis of this ECG? (2)
−15°.

What primary diagnosis can be made from this strip? (2)
This ECG is typical of the pre-excitation Wolff-Parkinson-White (WPW) syndrome. The minimum criteria for diagnosing the WPW syndrome are: a short PR (< 0.12 s) interval, a δ wave or initial slurring of the QRS complex and a QRS complex > 0.1 s in the presence of sinus rhythm.

What causes this condition? (2)
It is caused by an accessory bundle (the bundle of Kent) between the atria and ventricles which bypasses A-V conduction and causes a short PR interval and an abnormal spread

of ventricular depolarization. This anatomical pathway provides a potential for a re-entry tachyarrhythmia.

3. EQUIPMENT STATION

Commonly used equipment is often presented. This can involve the making up and explanation to an examiner of breathing systems (such as a Mapleson A system including the humidification device). You may be asked to explain the system or check it for safety features. Can you confidently check and demonstrate the safety features of a Bain circuit? Alternatively, you may go to an unmanned station and be asked questions.

Regarding the Entonox cylinder photographed below

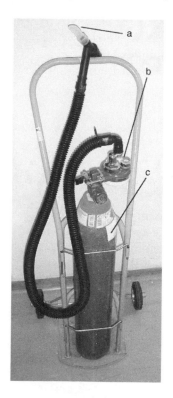

Label parts a, b and c. (1)
The parts are: (a) the mouth piece, (b) an on-demand valve
and (c) the cylinder.

What is in the cylinder? (2)
A mixture of 50% oxygen and 50% nitrous oxide.

What is its physical state? (2)
The mixture is in gaseous state. *Due to the Poynting Effect of
the gas admixture, nitrous oxide stays as a gas at or below its
critical temperature in spite of a cylinder pressure exceeding its
critical pressure.*

What is the pressure of a full cylinder? (1)
13700 kPa (137 bar or 2000 p.s.i.). *Use SI units when answering
questions.*

When half full, what is the pressure in the cylinder? (1)
Half of 13700 kPa = 6850 kPa.

What is the cylinder made of? (1)
Molybdenum steel.

What is the function of part b? (1)
It is a two-stage on-demand reducing valve.

Illustrate part b using a diagram. (5)

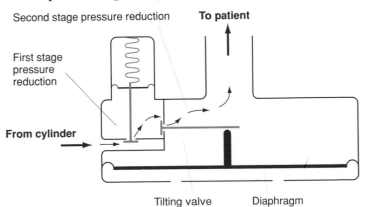

What is the critical temperature of Entonox? (1)
−5.5°C.

What is the critical temperature of oxygen? (1)
−118°C.

What is the critical temperature of nitrous oxide? (1)
36.5°C. *The critical temperature is the temperature above which a gas cannot be liquefied from the application of pressure alone. The pseudo-critical temperature is the critical temperature of a mixture of gases.*

Give one example of a clinical situation where the use of this system might be contraindicated. (1)
Pneumothorax *(air embolus, middle ear surgery are acceptable).*

Explain why? (2)
Expansion of air occurs. The reason for this is that N_2O is 34 times more soluble than nitrogen in blood, but because of partial pressure difference between N_2O in the blood and the air in the cavity, a larger quantity of N_2O will enter the cavity relative to the amount of nitrogen diffusing out.

4. SAFETY CHECK STATION

OSCE stations are used to confirm that the candidate has safe clinical principles from which to practise. Some stations such as the one below are simple but can have fatal consequences if done incorrectly. Don't be worried if you finish a station like this early. The examiner will relax you and have a chat if you have completed it after a couple of minutes.

Check this unit of blood and this patient in front of an examiner.

Two people are needed to check a unit of blood. Ask the examiner to check what you are doing as well. There may be an error in the form or the blood label.

- Name check with transfusion form (2)
- Ask to check the patient's identification band (patient and form the same?) (2)
- Confirm patient's date of birth (blood and form) (2)
- Confirm patient's hospital number (blood and form) (2)
- Ask patient name and date of birth if not anaesthetized (2)
- Confirm the blood unit number (2)
- Confirm the blood group and rhesus factor (2)
- What is the expiry date of the blood unit? (2)
- Is there any visible crack or tear in pack? (2)
- How long has pack been out of the blood refrigerator? (2)

5. RESUSCITATION STATION

The anaesthetist is the lynch pin of the 'cardiac arrest' team. In our experience, this station is marked quite severely. Often there is a practical side to it as well as a written short answer component and candidates have to work quickly. It should be routine.

Imagine that this mannequin is a person in ventricular fibrillation. Please defibrillate this mannequin using this defibrillator. (10)

There are essentially three controls (on, charge and discharge). Turn the machine on. Charge it up to 200 J for the initial defibrillation. Position the electrode gel pads correctly on the chest wall and order the examiner to stand back. Call 'stand clear' and check that everyone is clear. Don't wave the paddles around in the air. No paddles are allowed to touch ECG leads and glyceryl TNT patches. The oxygen supply is to be turned off during defibrillation to prevent an explosion. Discharge the device.

Please answer the following written questions about ventricular fibrillation.

What joules would you use for the first three consecutive defibrillations for a patient in ventricular fibrillation? (1)
200, 200 and 360 J.

What dose of amiodarone is used in cardiac arrest? (1)
300 mg.

How is it made up? (1)
With 20 ml 5% dextrose.

What is its indication for use? (1)
To treat shock refractory cardiac arrest due to pulseless ventricular tachycardia or ventricular fibrillation.

What further dose of amiodarone may be given? (1)
150 mg.

What is the infusion dose of amiodarone? (1)
1 mg/min for 6 h then 0.5 mg/min to a maximum of 2 g.

Can lidocaine be given to a patient who has received amiodarone? (1)
No.

What dose of magnesium can be used? (1)
8 mmol.

What is the indication for magnesium in ventricular fibrillation? (1)
To treat shock refractory ventricular fibrillation if the suspicion of hypomagnesaemia exists.

When is bicarbonate indicated at a cardiac arrest? (1)
A pH < 7.1 (hydrogen > 80 mmol/l).

6. CLINICAL MEASUREMENT QUESTION

Clinical measurement questions require detailed understanding and interpretation of the various investigations and monitoring that an anaesthetist performs both in theatre and in the intensive care unit. Normally the station is unmanned and a series of questions asked.

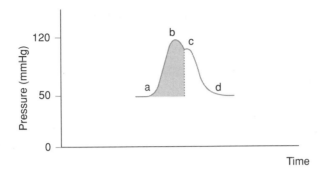

Look at this picture of an arterial pressure wave form and answer the following questions regarding it and pressure monitoring.

Name five properties of the pressure transducer system which prevent inaccuracies in the measurement of intra-arterial blood pressure. (10)

1. Non-compliant tubing
2. Short tubing
3. Non-dense fluid
4. No air bubbles in the fluid
5. Wide tubing

The natural frequency of the measuring apparatus is the frequency at which it resonates and amplifies the signal it receives. Therefore, to prevent amplification of the blood pressure signal, the natural frequency of the measuring system should be higher than 20 Hz which is the frequency of the blood pressure signal. The natural frequency is proportional to the diameter of the manometer tubing and inversely proportional to the density of the fluid inside the tubing and the square roots of both the tubing length and compliance.

Which letter represents the dichrotic notch? (2)
c.

What happens to the dichrotic notch if the systemic vascular resistance is low? (2)
The dichrotic notch is lowered. *(Slope 'cd' is also steeper.)*

What does slope 'ab' represent? (2)
Slope 'ab' is an index of contractility.

What happens to slope 'ab' in a patient with heart failure? (2)
It gets less steep.

What index of cardiac function does the shaded area represent? (2)
It is an index of stroke volume.

7. ANATOMY/LOCAL ANAESTHETIC BLOCK QUESTION

Only essential anatomy questions are likely to be asked. Unmanned stations will ask questions about a photograph or a drawing of a relevant piece of anatomy. Anatomy may also be asked in manned stations as part of a local anaesthetic technique question. It is fairly easy to anticipate any pure anatomy questions from knowing the common regional anaesthetic blocks that are performed. For example there may be an anatomy question on the brachial plexus. You may be asked to name it (roots, trunks, divisions, cords, nerves) and this would seem a fair question in lieu of the fact that brachial plexus blocks are commonly performed. Again a drawing of the femoral canal asking identification of labelled anatomical parts is reasonable.

Here is a drawing of an unlabelled anatomical structure. Please answer the following questions about it and about an anaesthetic technique related to this structure.

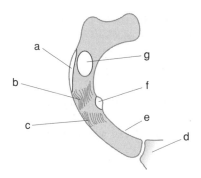

What is this structure? (1)
The first rib.

Identify the parts indicated by the labels a, b, c, d, e and f. (6)

a. Insertion of the serratus anterior muscle
b. The groove for the subclavian artery
c. The groove for the subclavian vein
d. The manubrium sternum
e. The scalenius medius muscle attachment point
f. The scalenius anterior muscle attachment point

Where does the brachial plexus pass over the first rib? (3)
It passes across the first rib behind the mid-point of the clavicle between the subclavian artery antero-medially and the scalenus medius muscle postero-laterally.

What attaches to edge g? (1)
Sibson's fascia (the supra-pleural membrane).

Regarding brachial plexus block:
Supraclavicular brachial plexus blockade runs the risk of which major complication? (1)
Pneumothorax *(haemothorax is acceptable)*.

Why? (2)
There is a close proximity between the first rib and the pleural dome.

Interscalene brachial plexus blockade can result in respiratory failure. List three causes of this? (3)

1. Accidental cerebrospinal fluid injection
2. Phrenic nerve palsy
3. Accidental pneumothorax

A block via the axillary route is likely to result in failure to block which nerve? (1)
The musculocutaneous nerve.

Axillary nerve blockade is not suitable for what operations on the upper limb? (2)
Operations on the shoulder.

8. DIAGNOSTIC/INTERPRETATION STATION

Chest X-rays, ECGs and scans are frequently read by anaesthetists, and a concise knowledge is expected. Occasionally angiograms relating to anatomy are asked. An example would be the arterial supply of the neck and head which is a reasonable question.

Look at this film and answer the following questions.

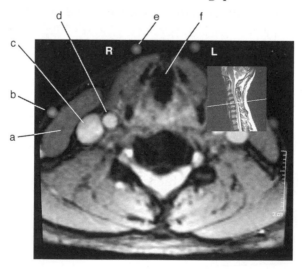

What is this film? (2)
This is a cervical MRI T2–weighted axial image showing the cross sectional anatomy of the neck at about C5.

Name the labelled structures. (6)

a. Sternocleidomastoid muscle
b. External jugular vein
c. Internal jugular vein
d. Carotid artery
e. Anterior jugular vein
f. Glottic opening

The internal jugular vein is the continuation of what vein? (2)
The sigmoid sinus.

The carotid sheath contains what three structures? (3)

1. The internal jugular vein
2. The vagus nerve
3. The carotid artery

What five factors favour cannulation of the internal jugular vein (IJV) on the right side (rather than the left side) of the neck? (5)

1. The right IJV is larger than the left and drains more blood from the cerebral hemispheres.
2. Its axis is more in line with the superior vena cava.
3. The thoracic duct which is present on the left side is susceptible to injury.
4. The pleural dome is lower on the right side.
5. Cannulation of the right IJV with palpation of the carotid pulse is technically easier for a right handed operator.

From which basal skull foramen does the internal jugular vein originate from? (2)
The jugular foramen at the base of the skull.

9. STATISTICS QUESTION

Every examination candidate dislikes statistics! Basically as a consultant or a specialist registrar you have to be able to read and understand scientific papers and research. There is a finite amount of basic statistics to understand. You will always be asked one statistics question in the OSCEs.

Please answer the following questions regarding statistical trials.

What is generally regarded as a significant '*p*' value? (2)
$p < 0.05$.

What does a *p* value of < 0.001 indicate? (2)
The observed difference will occur by chance once in a thousand times and is a highly significant value.

What test of statistical significance can be used for nominal, unpaired, non-parametric data? (2)
Chi-square test.

What test is commonly used for parametric data analysis? (2)
Student's *t* test.

What is a Type I error? (2)
A false positive result.

Look at the attached graphs and answer the following questions.

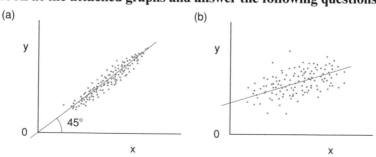

What is the regression equation for the line of best fit in figure 'a'? (2)
$y = x$.

Given that the regression equation for figure 'b' is $y = 1.2 + 0.4x$, state at which point would this line intercept the 'y' axis? (2)
1.2.

The graphs 'a' and 'b' have a similar number of points. Which line of best fit in these graphs should have a lower p value? (2)
Graph 'a.'

Why? (2)
Because the points in figure a are less dispersed. This is concluded visually from the figure.

What does a correlation coefficient of -1 indicate? (2)
It indicates a complete negative association.

10. COMMUNICATION SKILLS STATION

A 22–year-old primiparous pregnant patient wishes to know about pain relief in labour. She is particularly anxious about having epidural analgesia.

Introduce yourself and enquire as to the patient's general well being in pregnancy. Good morning. My name is Dr .... You look well. How has your health been in pregnancy? *I feel fine thanks – just heavy and fat. I have got a bit of backache at present.* You wish to see me about the methods of pain relief available to you in labour? (1) *Yes.*

There are several methods of pain relief available to you, I shall go through them for you. You should know that there are a small number of women who require no pain relief in labour. These are normally women who have had several babies and tend to have rapid deliveries (2). There are four common methods of analgesia available to women in labour.

About 70% of women use Entonox which is also called 'gas

and air.' It can be given to all women and provides pain relief effectively in early labour but must be used properly. As soon as a contraction is starting the gas must be inhaled. It does not affect the fetus but can make the mother feel sleepy and some-times nauseated (3). *My friend, Kylie, had that and she said it were useless.* Really, well let's talk about the other methods then.

About 50% of women use pethidine. This is an opiate which means it is like morphine. It is given intramuscularly and can be prescribed by the midwife looking after you. It can be given to all mothers but takes some 10–15 minutes to act. It is not a very good form of pain relief but it does make mothers feel relaxed and relieves a lot of the anxiety that they can have about the delivery. *Sounds great!* It can make the mother sleepy, nauseated, and can cause vomiting. *Will it affect my baby?* It can cross the placenta and affect the baby making it slow to breathe and sleepy so it is not given in the advanced stages of labour (3).

Epidural analgesia is given to a variable number of labour-ing women – about 30% in most busy units receive it. It is the best form of pain relief available. Most units now use a low dose mixture of drugs which provide good pain relief and allow the mother to remain mobile and she can walk with their birthing partner if she so wishes. Not everyone can have an epidural. If you don't want one you don't have to have one. Some mothers, especially those with pre-eclampsia, can have blood clotting abnormalities and this is a contraindication to an epidural. *Why? What's pre-eclampsia?* Why? Well, the epidural space has veins in it and if, whilst inserting the epidural, the anaesthetist hits one of these veins, they might bleed and not clot. This may lead to pressure being placed upon the spinal cord and lead to damage of the spinal cord which could be serious. Epidural analgesia must be safe and therefore it can't be done if the clotting is abnormal. We can check it is normal by a simple blood test. *Thanks.* Pre-eclamp-sia is high blood pressure, protein in the urine and swelling or oedema in pregnancy. That can be serious and it's why you have careful antenatal care. It needs careful treatment. *Oh! My friend Debra had that. She swelled up like a balloon and they done a caesarean on her. Her husband, Mike, well, he's a real mad Arsenal fan... goes to all the matches. Nice bloke... Feel sorry for her though... with him!* That's fascinating. I'm a Preston North End fan myself. *Who?* Pardon me?

Well, let's continue.

Any severe infection may be a contraindication and some mothers can be allergic to the drugs that are used (1).

An epidural is inserted by an experienced anaesthetist and new or inexperienced anaesthetists are not allowed to work in the delivery suite. Pain relief becomes effective within a couple of contractions and can be topped up by the midwife looking after you. Each top up lasts for about an hour. They have the advantage that they can be used if there are any complications in the labour – they can be used for caesarean sections, assisting forceps delivery or for retained placenta removal (4). There are some potential side effects that can happen. The main one that can affect the patient is that of headache. This affects less than one in 100 patients in most units but it can be severe and will, in the worst cases, make you lie in bed and make it difficult for you to look after your baby. It can be cured but will slow your recovery down for a few days after the delivery.

Once the epidural is inserted the midwife will need to monitor your blood pressure regularly whilst the epidural is being topped up and you will need an intravenous drip. Epidurals are associated with an increased incidence of forceps deliveries but there is no evidence that they cause them. Delivery and pregnancy cause backache often but there is no evidence that the incidence of backache is higher in those mothers who have had an epidural. A correctly sited and managed epidural does not cause paralysis either but this is often what women worry about so you can be reassured on this point too (4).

Finally some mothers use transcutaneous nerve stimulators – TENS machines – which are electrical devices which are attached to the back and provide a pleasant tingling sensation which helps counter the pain of the contraction. Acupuncture is also used occasionally (1). These techniques are really only successful in early labour but have no side effects.

I hope this discussion answers your anxieties. Any questions? (1)

Questions asked during the discussion by the patient may include: When will I get normal sensation again after the 'epidural'? Do 'epidurals' slow down labour? How likely am I to have a caesarean?

II. MONITORING DEVICE QUESTION

Common topics are commonly asked. Occasionally a topic is so important that it can come up in all parts of the examination. Capnography can be asked in vivas, MCQs and in the OSCEs. A fundamental knowledge of the traces is required. Do you know how a capnograph works?

Look at the drawing of the attached capnography traces and answer the following questions.

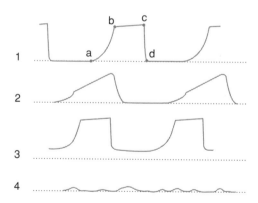

On trace 1 where is the start of inspiration? (2)
Point 'c.'

On trace 1 where is the start of expiration? (2)
Point 'a.'

Explain the shapes of line 'ab.'(2)
Line 'ab' represents the start of expiration – dead space gas initially with an increasing amount of alveolar gas added as point 'b' is approached.

Explain the shape of line 'bc.'(2)
Line 'bc' represents an almost horizontal line (plateau) due to the expiration of predominantly alveolar gas.

What is the abnormality in trace 2? (2)
A slowly rising expiratory slope of CO_2 excretion with no plateau.

Name two examples of clinical conditions that would give such a trace. (2)
This is characteristic of airway obstruction. Examples include asthma and chronic obstructive airway disease.

What is the abnormality in trace 3? (2)
Rebreathing of CO_2.

List four possible causes. (2)

a. A fresh gas flow below the critical rebreathing level for the type of breathing system used
b. Expiring or expired soda lime
c. Malfunctioning one-way valve or APL valve
d. A large apparatus dead space

Describe trace 4. (1)
There is no or very little CO_2 production

List three possible reasons for this. (3)

1. Technical. Occlusion of the sampling line, disconnection of the circuit
2. Cardiac. Cardiac arrest, very low cardiac output
3. Respiratory. Oesophageal intubation, accidental extubation

12. ANATOMY

Know your basic anatomy! Questions on pure anatomy are easy if you have learnt it and impossible if you haven't. This is a difficult question.

Look at this picture of the base of the skull.

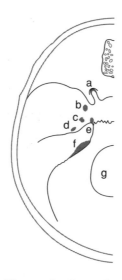

Name the foramina labelled a-g. (7)

a. Optic foramen
b. Foramen rotundum
c. Foramen ovale
d. Foramen spinosum
e. Foramen lacerum
f. Jugular foramen
g. Foramen magnum

What important structures pass through these foramina? (7)

a. Optic nerve and vessels
b. Maxillary branch of the Vth cranial nerve
c. Mandibular branch of Vth cranial nerve

d. Middle meningeal artery
e. Internal carotid
f. Jugular vein
g. Spinal cord

What two structures pass through the cribiform plate? (2)

1. Olfactory nerves
2. Dural extension with cerebrospinal fluid

The spinal cord in an adult ends at the lower border of what vertebra? (2)
The first lumbar vertebra.

Through what is cerebrospinal fluid absorbed back into the circulation? (2)
The sigmoid venous sinuses.

13. TECHNICAL SKILLS QUESTION

In front of an examiner and with an actor or a model the candidate can be asked to explain how a local anaesthetic block or a practical procedure might be performed. This done for two reasons. Firstly anaesthetists perform blocks on awake patients and have to be able to explain what they are doing to the patients and secondly anaesthetists have to be able to teach others and explain the relevant technique.

This station is about cannulation of the internal jugular vein. A model or dummy is present. It has various labels on it. Identify the labels a–f. (6)

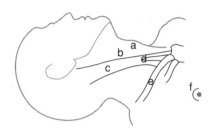

a. Thyroid cartilage
b. Carotid artery pulsation *(you can visualize it and palpate it on the dummy in reality)*
c. Sternocleidomastoid muscle (SCM) with its anterior (medial) border and posterior (lateral) border
d. Apex of the triangle formed by the sternal and clavicular heads of the muscle
e. The point between the medial and middle thirds of the clavicle
f. Ipsilateral nipple

Describe and show how you would perform cannulation of the internal jugular vein on this dummy? (10)
I wish to obtain patient consent.

I wish to exclude any contraindications, in particular those relating to bleeding disorders. I need to know if the patient is on drugs like warfarin or has any disease that can interfere with clotting. There appears to be no anatomical abnormalities such as an enlarged thyroid which will interfere with the procedure.

The procedure needs to be carried out under strict aseptic conditions. I can ensure asepsis by hand scrubbing, wearing a sterile gown and gloves, preparing the skin with chlorhexidine, and by covering the chest and head with sterile drapes.

I shall place the patient in the supine position with a 15–20° head-down tilt to increase venous return and jugular vein filling. This also reduces the risk of air embolism.

I shall adjust the shoulders and extend the arms alongside the body to achieve symmetry of the upper chest and neck. I can extend the neck by placing a towel roll under the shoulders and shall turn the head to the opposite side. This is usually the left side as I preferentially select the right internal jugular vein (IJV) to cannulate.

I also find it useful to identify the jugular venous waves. I can distinguish them from arterial pulsations by close inspection whilst feeling the arterial pulse or listening to the beat of the pulse oximeter. I can ballot the IJV in this case too.

I can use one of two approaches for cannulation of the internal jugular vein *[these are illustrated below. Lateral and anterior line-draw views are used to show the angles to the coronal and sagittal (median) planes, respectively]*.

I use the high anterior approach 'a' in most cases. The point of insertion of the needle is chosen at the medial border of the SCM at the level of superior border or the prominence of the thyroid cartilage, or at the SCM mid-point along its course between the origin and insertion of the muscle. The carotid pulse is palpated. This is to ensure the needle is entered lateral to the artery. Directions of the needle are an angle of 30–40° to the coronal plane and 10–30° to the sagittal plane. The ipsilateral nipple or the point between the medial and middle thirds of the clavicle can also be used to adjust for the angle with the sagittal plane.

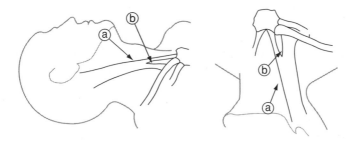

The lower apex approach 'b' is an alternative technique which I find particularly useful when the carotid pulsation is difficult to palpate. This carries a higher risk of pneumothorax as a complication. The SCM and the triangle formed by its sternal and clavicular heads are identified. The needle is inserted in the apex of the triangle in a direction of 30–45° to the coronal plane and 0–10° to the sagittal plane. The vein is entered about 1–3 cm from the skin.

I prefer to use a 'needle through needle' device to perform the cannulation. A wire can be passed once the vein is punctured. I aspirate on the syringe whilst entering the vein.

Name four major complications of central venous cannulation. (4)
1. Pneumothorax
2. Carotid artery puncture
3. Air embolus
4. Nerve damage (vagus, phrenic)

14. HISTORY TAKING STATION

This station is simply about doing exactly what you do before every anaesthetic. The only problem here is that you have a finite amount of time to take the history so you must be very focused. The easiest way to do this station is to ask specific questions about the anaesthetic and operation and then perform a more general anaesthetic review. The examiners mark in this way also. Think about what might have caused the need for this operation. A cholecystectomy can be done for a variety of reasons; stones, cholecystitis or pancreatitis. The operation may be more difficult if there are complications arising from the pancreatitis. Similarly a person with a fractured neck of femur may have a pathological fracture, tripped and fallen, or had a syncopal episode from a Stokes Adams attack.

A 25–year-old man presents for a knee arthroscopy in the day care unit. He has told the pre-admission nurse that when he had his appendix removed he awoke in the Intensive Care Unit but knows nothing else. Take an anaesthetic history.

(Specific questions first)

Introduce yourself, identify the patient, the operation and the consent. Good morning. My name is Dr .... You are having a knee arthroscopy? *Yes.* Which side? *The left.* Is it marked? *Yes.* I'll show you. Have you signed your consent form? *Yes.* You once had your appendix removed and woke up in the ITU? (2) *That's right. (Questioning should now relate to this operation.)* Regarding your appendix removal – was the operation completed as scheduled? (2) *Yes. They said it was an anaesthetic problem. The anaesthetist was very young but that's all I know. I remember him being very upset. I moved down to London after that.* When and where did you have this operation? (1) ... I'll write and get the notes from that hospital. You obviously have no knowledge of what happened but we need to try to find out what happened so I am going to ask you some questions relating to this incident. Have you only had one anaesthetic? *No. I had an arthroscopy one year before the appendix job.* Were there any problems with that anaesthetic? (1) *No.* Were you investigated or asked to return for investigations after your appendix operation? (1) *They did some blood tests I think but I never got the results because I moved to London.* Are you allergic to any drugs? (1) *No.*

Has anyone in your family had any anaesthetic problems? *No.* Has anyone ever been admitted to the Intensive Care Unit after an operation or anaesthetic? (1) *Hold on, my dad said he'd been in ITU once but I don't know why?* Is there any family history of temperature abnormalities in anaesthesia? (1) *No.* Do any family members carry Medic-alert bracelets or cards warning of risks with anaesthesia or from drugs? (1) *No.* Do you vomit easily, have a history of reflux or indigestion? (1) *No.* Thank you. You've answered all my specific questions about that. I'll ask some other questions now.

(General questions second)

Are you on any drugs normally? (1) *No.* How much do you smoke and drink? *I don't.* Any sputum? (1) *None!* Do you have any medical illnesses? (1) *No.* Specifically do you have any heart or lung disease, hypertension, diabetes or any illnesses? (1) *No.* Do you have any loose or false teeth or any caps or crowns? (1) *No.* When did you last eat or drink? (1) *Last night.* Thank you. Do you wish to add any thing else? *No. I'm starving. When's my 'op' Doc?*

The examiner will now ask you if you would anaesthetize him today? You wouldn't. You suspect he has pseudocholinesterase deficiency and will need blood testing before any operation (2).

15. DIAGNOSTIC/RADIOLOGY QUESTION

The diagnosis, investigations, and management of several condi-tions, especially trauma, is important. Trauma is asked in all parts of the examination. Try this question.

A 20-year-old male was brought to casualty with multiple injuries. He received initial resuscitation and investigations. Part of his investigations included the film printed below. Please answer the following questions about this film and patient.

What is this radiological film? (1)
CT scan of the brain.

What are the four abnormal radiological findings? (4)
The findings are: left extradural haematoma, obliterated posterior horn of the lateral ventricle, midline shift and large scalp haematoma.

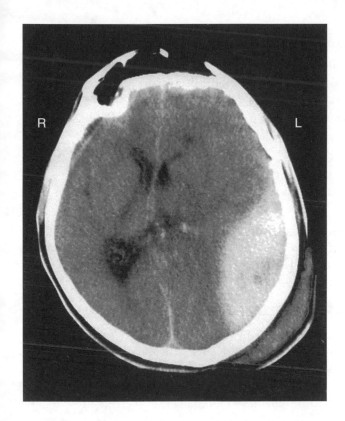

What is the cause of the extradural haematoma? (2)
Rupture of the middle meningeal artery. *Less commonly it can be caused by ruptured sagittal or transverse sinuses.*

What is the normal intracranial pressure? (1)
7–15 mmHg.

There is a risk of tentorial herniation in this patient. Why? (2)
This is evident from the obvious increased pressure and visible midline shift.

Which nerve(s) is/are responsible for the pupillary dilatation? (2)
The oculomotor (III cranial) nerve is responsible.

Would you expect pupillary dilatation to develop on the right side? Why? (2)
No. It is expected on the left side. Nerve pressure will develop on the same side as the haematoma.

What nerve supplies the lateral rectus muscle? (1)
The VIth cranial (abducens) nerve.

What nerve supplies the medial rectus muscle? (1)
The IIIrd cranial (oculomotor) nerve.

What nerves are tested for in the pupillary light reflex test? (4)
The afferent arc is the optic (II) nerve and the efferent arc is the oculomotor (III) nerve.

16. ANATOMY QUESTION

This question is added in case you thought that as there is likely to be only one anatomy question you can fail it and still pass. Anatomy comes into many questions and there is often more than one. You need to know this question because you perform regional anaesthesia, especially epidural anaesthesia, on patients.

Here is a picture illustrating three vertebrae. They are labelled a, b and c. Answer the following questions about them.

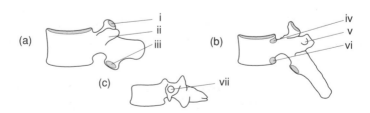

Name the regions of the vertebral column to which the vertebrae a, b and c belong? (3)

a. Lumbar
b. Thoracic
c. Cervical

What are the features that differentiate between them? (6)

a. The lumbar region has large vertebral bodies which are horizontal and relatively short with wide spinous processes.
b. The thoracic region has relatively small vertebral bodies with long oblique spinous processes. There are also differentiated by having articular surfaces (or demi-facets) on the body of vertebrae and their transverse processes which are for the heads and tubercles of the ribs, respectively.
c. The main differential features of the cervical vertebrae are that they have transversarium foramina and cloven spinous processes.

Label the parts indicated by i, ii, iii, iv, v, vi and vii. (7)

i   Superior articular process
ii   Transverse process
iii Inferior articular process
iv   Superior demi-facet for rib head
v   Articular process for rib tubercle
vi   Inferior demi-facet for rib head
vii Transversarium foramen

Which vertebra has no vertebral body? (1)
The atlas.

On which vertebra is the odontoid peg found? (1)
The second cervical vertebra (axis).

Which structures pass through the transversarium foramen? (2)
The vertebral arteries.

OSCE Examination B

I. CLINICAL EXAMINATION STATION

Examine this 22-year-old man's respiratory system.

A patient is lying on an examination table. After introducing yourself, explain what you are going to do. Similar topics include examination of the cardiovascular system and the cranial nerves. An examiner is present at this station. You do not have to talk to the examiner but it is sensible to explain what you are doing and looking for.

Good morning. My name is Dr .... I'm going to examine your respiratory system (1).

His general appearance indicates that he looks well. There is no evidence of anaemia when I look at the mucosa under his lower eyelid. Put your tongue out please. It is normal. His breathing is 12/min and regular and he has a normal pattern of respiration (1).

May I look at your hands? I can see some tar staining from nicotine on his fingers. There is no clubbing. His nails are normal as are his palms (2).

Let me look at your neck and chest now. The pattern of respiration is normal. There is no evidence of an obstructive or a restrictive pattern of breathing. His lips are not pursed and there is no accessory muscle use, as judged from looking at his neck (2).

Let me closely examine your neck. There are no nodes to be felt. Could you lie down now. I shall raise the bed head a little. Please look away from me. *I am looking for the jugular venous pulse.* Breathe in. Hold it and breathe out and hold it. Breathe normally. *The jugular venous pressure is low and within normal limits (2).*

I now need to inspect your chest from in front of you and from behind. Sit forward please. The rate is 12/min. The shape of the chest is normal. There are no scars or nodules. There is symmetrical chest wall expansion (3).

May I feel your chest and neck? On palpation the trachea is midline. The apex beat can be palpated at the left fifth intercostal space 10 cm from the sternal edge. Say '99'. *'99'.*

Vocal fremitus is normal. I can feel no lymph nodes in the axillae (3).
When I percuss the chest it is resonant and normal all over.
I have compared both sides of the chest at the front and back.
The heart appears not to be enlarged (3).
I wish to listen to your chest. *Use the diaphragm of the stethoscope to auscultate the chest.* The breath sounds are normal in nature and intensity all over the chest. There is normal vocal resonance (3).
This man's respiratory system examination is normal. *(I hope!)*

2. ANAESTHETIC MACHINE CHECK

This is fundamental to both the examination and safe anaesthetic practice. Check the anaesthetic machine routinely as part of your routine practice. This station should be passed by every candidate. There are guidelines from the Association of Anaesthetists' of Great Britain and Ireland and these should be the basis of the check list. An examiner has a check list from which he will mark you. You need to explain what you are doing to the examiner.

Similar questions relate to safety of breathing and circle systems. Make sure you understand what an APL valve pressure of 60 cmH₂O means.

Check the safety features on this anaesthetic machine (no breathing circuit, ventilator, monitoring equipment or ancillary equipment are present).
Is there an electrical supply to the machine? Is it turned on? (1)
Is an oxygen analyser present? Is it switched on? Is it calibrated? (2) *Make sure you know how to calibrate the analyzer.*
Are there pipeline gases? Are they connected? Can you perform a 'tug test' on the pipes? Is there correct connection of the pipes to the appropriate gas supply? (2)
Ensure that there is not a carbon dioxide cylinder attached to the machine (1). *If there is, remove it.* Check that there are,

ideally, two nitrous oxide and oxygen cylinders attached (1). If there is only one of each ensure that spares are present. Check for Bodok seals (1). Are blanking plugs fitted to the empty yokes? (1) Check the pressures. Is the pipeline pressure 400 kPa? (2) What are the cylinder pressures? *Remember a full oxygen cylinder is 13 700 kPa and a full nitrous oxide cylinder is 5400 kPa. Do you know how the pressures change in these cylinders as they empty?* How full are these cylinders? (2) Check the flow meter function. Are the valves smooth and bobbins free? (2) Does the emergency bypass for oxygen work? *What is the flow rate of oxygen through it?* Is there an oxygen failure alarm? Is it possible to give a hypoxic mixture? (2) Are the vaporizers filled? Are they seated correctly? Are there O-rings present? Any leaks in the vaporizers? (2) Is there a scavenging system present? (1)

3. HISTORY TAKING STATION

A 35-year-old lady presents for an elective laparoscopic cholecystectomy. Take a history from her.

There is always a history taking station in every OSCE examination. Some history taking stations occur which, as in real life, are devoid of patient problems. Remember specific and general questioning is necessary.

(Specific)

Introduce yourself. Identify the patient and the operation. Check consent. Good afternoon. My name is Dr .... You are having your gall bladder removed? *Yes.* Have you signed this consent form I see here? (1) *Yes.* Why are you having a cholecystectomy? (2) *A what?* Sorry. Your gall bladder out? *I got infection from stones that are in it.* How did the disease initially present? (2) *Pain, vomiting and they admitted me to hospital for 5 days.* So, how long have you had gall bladder disease? (1) *I've known about it 5 months now. I've been on the waiting list 3 months but I've still been getting pain on and off.* Thank you.

(General)

Do you normally take any drugs? (1) *Medicinal or recreational? No. I take Arnica because I bruise easily and Cod Liver Oil capsules to stop the pain.* Oh! Do you have any allergies? (1) *Doctors! Hospitals! Winter! Arsenal! Ha, ha, ha!* Good joke but I meant drug allergies. *Yes. Penicillin.* What happens? *I don't know. I was a child when it happened.* Thank you. Do you drink alcohol? (1) *Wine at the weekends. Not much though.* Do you smoke? Do you cough up any sputum? (1) *No.* Have you had any previous operations? *Yes.* What were they? (1) *My wisdom teeth were taken out 10 years ago.* Any troubles with the anaesthetic? (2) *Not that I know of.* Has any member of your family had anaesthetic difficulties? (1) *No.*

Have you a history of any illnesses? (1) *Migraine sometimes but nothing else.* Specifically do you have any history of hypertension, tuberculosis, diabetes, or heart disease? (1) *No.* Do you suffer from gastric indigestion of reflux? *Now and then.* How severe is it? (1) *It's not really a problem at all.*

Do you have any dentures, caps, crowns or loose teeth? (1) *Yes. I've got three on my upper front teeth. They're fixed though.* Are you starved? *Starving more like! Ha, ha, ha.* When did you last eat? (1) *Last night.* When did you last drink? (1) *Three hours ago.* Thank you.

4. ELECTROCARDIOGRAPH DIAGNOSTIC STATION

Read the following electrocardiograph and answer the following questions.

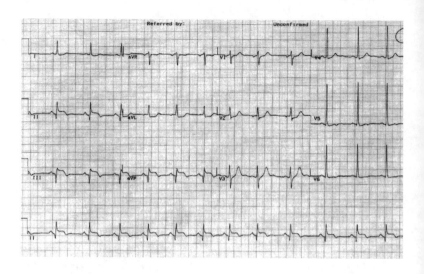

What is the heart rate? (2)
75

What is the axis? (2)
+9°

Is this axis abnormal? (2)
This is a normal axis (−30° to +90°).

What are the abnormalities in this trace? (2)
Q waves and ST elevation in leads II, III and aVF.

What diagnosis can be inferred from this electrocardiograph? (2)
Inferior myocardial infarction.

What is the blood supply to the interventricular septum? (2)
The left anterior descending artery.

What is the width of a normal QRS complex? (2)
It is less than 0.12 s (three small squares).

What component of the cardiac muscle action potential does the T wave represent? (2)
Ventricular repolarization.

What is the PR interval in this trace? (2)
140 ms.

What is the blood supply to the SA node in the majority of people? (2)
The right coronary artery.

5. DATA ANALYSIS QUESTION

This is an unmanned station. You just have to fill in the answers from a clinical scenario. Remember to learn definitions including those of clinical situations. Do you know a sensible definition of respiratory failure and malignant hyperthermia? What is the P50?

A 20-year-old male has been brought to the hospital after a road traffic accident. He, apparently, has injuries mainly to his pelvic region. On examination, he is noted to have some bruises to his lower abdomen but no open wounds. He is described as restless and cold.

During his assessment in casualty the following observations are noted; pulse 125/min, arterial pressure 80/40 and respiratory rate 32/min. X-rays shows a fractured pelvis and a fractured femur.

Arterial sample for blood gas analysis on room air gives the following results:

pH 7.19, PaO_2 13.6 kPa, $PaCO_2$ 3.4 kPa, HCO_3 9.9 and SBE –12.

Answer the following questions.

What is the normal $PaO2$ in a healthy 20-year-old breathing air? (2)
About 13 kPa.

If he were being given 60% oxygen through a fixed performance mask what would you expect the PaO_2 to be? (2)
About 50 kPa. *The alveolar gas equation needs to be applied here.* $PaO_2 = P_IO_2 - PaCO_2/R$ *where* R *is the respiratory quotient.*

A pH of 7.4 is equal to how many hydrogen ions in nmol/l? (2)
40.

What does this acid-base picture show? (2)
It is metabolic acidosis. *There is a low HCO_3 and there is a base deficit.*

Why has this metabolic picture arisen? (2)
There is hypoperfusion, as a result of hypovolaemia, from the haemorrhage.

Explain the $PaCO_2$. (2)
It is low due to compensatory hyperventilation.

What is the normal level of $PaCO_2$? (2)
About 5.3 kPa.

What is the normal range of HCO_3? (2)
20–24 mmol/l.

Define 'standard bicarbonate concentration'. (2)
'Standard bicarbonate concentration' is the concentration of bicarbonate in the plasma from blood which is equilibrated with a gas with a PCO_2 of 5.3 kPa. As PCO_2 is controlled, it is thus a measure of metabolic bicarbonate.

Define 'standard base excess'. (2)
'Standard base excess' is the base excess value calculated for anaemic blood (haemoglobin = 5 g/dl). *The rationale of this is that this closely represents the* in vivo *buffering capacity of the whole human body because in the interstitial fluid there is no haemoglobin and less protein.*

6. CLINICAL ANATOMY STATION

Demonstrating blocks and anatomy on models to an examiner is to be expected. Sometimes there is a clinical content to them such as in this question.

Show where the nerves of the wrist and elbow are in this patient. Explain how they may become damaged in anaesthesia.

Good morning. My name is Dr .... May I see your wrist please? At the wrist lie the three nerves that supply the hand (2). On the anterior aspect of the wrist lie the ulnar and the median nerves (2). Please flex your wrist. Thank you. Flexing the wrist has shown me the tendon of palmaris longus and lateral to it you can see flexor digitorum communis. Between these tendons lies the median nerve (2). The ulnar nerve lies lateral to the tendon of flexor carpi ulnaris and medial to the pulsatile ulnar artery which I can feel here (1). Turn your wrist around. The branches of the radial artery fan out over the posterior aspect of the wrist (1). These nerves are most likely to be damaged from pressure especially when the patient is in the prone position with the wrists dangling over the arm supports. Venous and arterial cannulation attempts may also damage the ulnar nerve (2).

Please may I look at your elbow? At the elbow the ulnar nerve lies posteriorly and lateral to the ulnar styloid (2). It can be damaged from direct pressure whilst the patient is in the supine position especially if arm supports are not padded to stop direct nerve pressure (2). The radial nerve lies laterally as it passes out of its humeral grove and is similarly at risk (2). The median nerve lies here. It is deep within the antecubital fossa and medial to the brachial artery (2). It can be damaged directly by puncture from needles. Drugs can also damage it, for example, in thiopentone extravasation (2).

Thank you.

7. RESUSCITATION STATION

There are often two examiners at this station. There is an observer too and a formidable amount of resuscitation equipment around. It is often daunting. There are mannequins and various pieces of resuscitation apparatus. Remember to learn paediatric as well as adult resuscitation. Remember to learn the management of choking as well as the management of the three arrest arrhythmias: ventricular fibrillation, pulseless electrical activity and asystole. You are often asked to fill in the gaps of the algorithms.

Demonstrate 'Basic Life Support' on this adult mannequin assuming it to be an unresponsive patient.
Check the patient's responsiveness – *ask* 'Are you all right?'. *Call* 'Help!'*(2). Open the airway – *clear it, apply head tilt, and lift the chin (2).*

Now check the breathing – *look, listen, feel. Say* 'if this patient were breathing and had no evidence of a head injury I would place him in the recovery position' (2). Give the patient two effective breaths (2). *Use an anaesthetic mask and bag if they are present and available. If they are not you will have to give effective mouth to mouth resuscitation. Practise it before the examination!*

Assess the circulation and check for the pulse - *10 s only - the carotid pulse is an acceptable pulse for anaesthetists to palpate. (You can feel no pulse.) State* 'If there were a circulation in this situation I would continue rescue breathing and check the circulation every minute but there isn't. I need to apply chest compressions appropriately (2).

Compress the chest at rate 100/min and in a ratio of compression to breathing of 15: 2. Remember to apply the compressions in the right place using correct hand positions. You must know this. Keep breathing the mannequin and applying chest compressions until asked to stop (6).

Tell me *(the examiner)* the potentially reversible causes of cardiac arrest. (4)
The causes of potentially reversible cardiac arrest are four Hs and four Ts. These are:

• Hypoxia

- Hypovolaemia
- Hyper/hypokalaemia
- Hypothermia
- Tension pneumothorax
- Tamponade (cardiac)
- Toxic/therapeutic disorders
- Thromboembolic or mechanical obstruction

Thank you.

8. ANATOMY AND LOCAL ANAESTHETIC BLOCK STATION

A model of the ankle is present. The station is manned by an examiner. Describe to him the anatomy of the nerves to the foot as they pass the ankle. Describe how you would do an ankle block to him.
Hello.

The nerves to the ankle are five in number. Four are derived from the sciatic nerve. These are the tibial, sural, deep peroneal and superficial peroneal nerves. The other nerve is derived from the terminal branch of the femoral nerve, and is named the saphenous nerve (3). Two nerves at the ankle lie posteriorly. These are the tibial and sural nerves. The others lie anteriorly (2).

I'm going to tell and show you about these nerves individually. *That's fine by me.*

The sural nerve supplies the heel and the posterior half of the foot. It passes the ankle superficially lateral to the tendon Achilles. *Point to it.* It is blocked by passing a 22 gauge, 3 cm needle using an aseptic technique lateral to the tendon Achilles at a level just superior to the lateral malleolus. About 5–7 ml of a non-adrenaline containing local anaesthetic needs to be given (3).

The tibial nerve lies medial to the tendon Achilles and lateral to the posterior tibial artery. *Palpate it.* Here it is. It supplies the anterior aspect of the sole of the foot and the bottoms of the toes. A 22 gauge needle passed here at the cephalad border of the medial malleolus will provide suitable blockade of this nerve with 5 ml of local anaesthetic solution (3).

The top of the foot is supplied by fan like branches from the other three nerves. The saphenous nerve lies medially at a superficial level, the deep peroneal nerve lies here, immediately lateral to the pulse of the anterior tibial artery *(palpate it)* at the level of the superior level of the medial malleolus, and the superficial peroneal nerve lies laterally at a subcutaneous level (3). The nerves can be blocked by the insertion of a 22 gauge needle lateral to the anterior tibial artery pulse and injecting 3 ml of local anaesthetic agent here. I would then inject subcutaneously medially and laterally to block the other nerves. Five ml of local anaesthetic needs to be fanned out in each direction (4).

The dose of local anaesthetic must not exceed toxicity and with bupivacaine this is 2 mg/kg. In an average person about 20 ml of 0.375% could be used in total for the block (1).

What does the word 'one percent' mean? (1)
1 g per 100 ml which is 10 mg/ml.

Well done. We've finished this early. Where do you work? Northwick Park Hospital, Sir. *Oh. I know it well.*

9. MEASUREMENT QUESTION

You need to know and understand the basic traces that you see every day. You need to be able to explain them.

This station requires you to draw a wave form pattern and then answer some questions.

Draw a central venous pressure trace showing the normal waveform configuration.

Label all the waves and descents. (6)

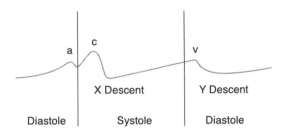

There are three waves. Explain the source of each wave. (3)

- The 'a' wave is a positive deflection caused by atrial contraction.
- The 'c' wave represents the initial bulging of the tricuspid valve into the atrium with the onset of ventricular contraction. The adjacent pulse of the carotid artery also makes a contribution, hence the name 'c' wave.
- The 'v' wave is a positive deflection that occurs as blood accumulates in the vena cavae and right atrium whilst the tricuspid valve is closed.

There are two descents. Explain each descent. (3)

- The 'x' descent follows as the atrium relaxes and the tricuspid valve is pulled downward during ventricular contraction.
- The 'y' descent results from opening of the tricuspid valve and the start of right ventricular filling.

What characteristic wave form changes may be seen or expected in each of the following abnormalities?

Atrial fibrillation. (2)
An absence of 'a' wave.

Complete heart block. (2)
There are giant 'a' waves or 'cannon' waves which may be seen when the atrium contracts against a closed tricuspid valve.

Tricuspid regurgitation. (2)
There is an absence of 'x' descent with a large c-v wave. *There is a rise of right atrial pressure due to the regurgitation of blood during ventricular contraction.*

Tricuspid stenosis. (2)
A large 'a' wave amplitude may be seen due to the atrium contracting against an increased resistance.

10. COMMUNICATION SKILLS STATION

An examiner is present with a patient. You will be required to explain some aspect of anaesthetic care to her. Some actresses are 'aggressive' with the candidate. This lady is benign. Similar subjects may include an explanation of awake fibre-optic intubation to a very anxious lady, entering patients into clinical drug trials, and explaining absent dentition after an operation.

This is Mrs Hasan. She is a 35-year-old lady, pregnant with twins, who is about to undergo her first elective caesarean section. Discuss the methods of anaesthesia available to her for this operation.
Introduce yourself, identify the patient and check the consent.
Good afternoon. My name is Dr .... You are going to have a caesarean section? *Yes.* Have you signed your consent? (1) *Yes.* You wish to discuss the techniques of anaesthesia available to you? *Oh! Yes please.*
   Anaesthesia for caesarean section can be delivered by two methods. These are regional or general anaesthesia (1). *Pardon?* Sorry! I mean general anaesthesia or local anaesthetic techniques. Each method has advantages and disadvantages and I shall tell you about each technique.
   Let's talk about regional anaesthesia first. About 90% of elective caesarean sections are performed using this method. Some mothers think that they will be unable to cope with the fear and anxiety of being awake in this situation but almost all mothers prefer it once the block is established (1). The advantages are that this is a safer technique for both you and the

babies, the babies receive no anaesthetic, you will be awake for the birth of your children, your husband or birthing partner will be able to be present and supportive of you, you recover more quickly, you do not suffer from any of the risks or side effects of general anaesthesia, and we are able to provide you with better postoperative analgesia (2). The disadvantages are that there is a real risk, albeit very small, of a headache which can be severe. If this happens it will slow your recovery down for a few days. We can treat it well though (2). Occasionally the block cannot be performed or does not work perfectly. I shall check the block before surgery starts to ensure that this has not happened but in a very small percentage of patients general anaesthesia has to be considered because the block is inadequate (2).

I shall require that you and I work as a team – I shall get you into a position so that the block can be performed and I need you to stay still so that I can perform the block safely. I prefer to do it with you sitting up (2). *Great! I feel faint if I lie down.*

General anaesthesia is normally done because of the patient's preference for it and we respect the right for the patient to have an influence on the decision making (1). The advantage of general anaesthesia is that the patient is asleep (2). There are many disadvantages in this elective situation – the risks and side effects of general anaesthesia are real – nausea, drowsiness, and vomiting occur afterwards and it is more difficult to provide you with excellent postoperative analgesia. Your husband will not be able to be present and you will obviously not be aware when the babies are born (2). The anaesthetic can pass through the placenta and make the babies more sleepy initially but this is not normally a problem and there are special baby doctors present to deal with any difficulties that they might encounter (2).

On balance, as you can tell I favour you to be awake for the operation and I'm sure that it will be a rewarding and fulfilling experience for you (2). Any questions? *No. That's fine.*

Questions that may be asked by a different patient include: How will I know that I will not be awake if I have to be put to sleep?

How long will I be numb for afterwards? When will I be able to eat? How soon can I breast feed? Will the anaesthetic pass into the mother's milk? What is a spinal anaesthetic? How does it differ from an epidural?

11. CHEST X-RAY DIAGNOSIS AND INVESTIGATION

An unmanned station with an X-ray and several questions requiring answers can be present.

Look at this X-ray. Answer the following questions.

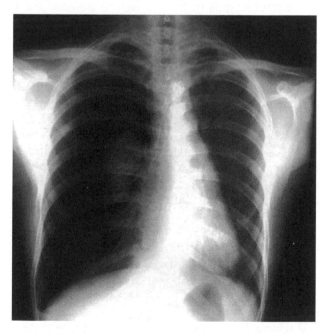

What is the cardio-thoracic ratio in this X-ray? (2)
0.45.

Is this within normal limits? (2)
Yes. The normal limit is less than 0.5.

How can you tell if the X-ray is centrally positioned? (2)
Symmetrical clavicles and scapulae position.

In a normal chest X-ray which hemi-diaphragm is higher? Why? (2)
The right because it is elevated from below by the liver.

What are the four abnormal findings on this chest X-ray? (4)
1. Absence of lung parenchymal markings on the right side
2. Retracted lung margins in the right hilar region
3. A shift of upper mediastinum and heart shadow to the left
4. Mediastinal air visible

What is the diagnosis? (2)
The diagnosis is tension pneumothorax with pneumomediastinum.

List four clinical signs expected to be found in this condition? (4)
The clinical signs include: tachypnoea, difficulty in breathing, reduced chest expansion and increased resonance on the right side, reduced breath sounds on the same side and shift of the trachea to the opposite (left) side which may be palpated in the suprasternal region. Additionally, in tension pneumothorax the high intrathoracic pressure reduces venous return leading to a reduction in cardiac output and hypotension.

What intervention might this condition require? (2)
This is a life-threatening emergency. Initially, release of the intrapleural air can be achieved rapidly and effectively by inserting a cannula in the second intercostal space at the mid-clavicular line. Subsequently, an intrapleural chest drain can be inserted into the sixth intercostal space at the mid-axillary line and connected to a one-way valve or an underwater seal.

12. STATISTICS QUESTION

A basic statistics question is always present. Don't ignore this subject! The station is unmanned and requires answers to questions.

Draw a Normal distribution curve. (2) Draw lines for 1 and 2 standard deviations on either sides of the mean on it. (2) Write down the proportions of data that would lie within these lines. (2)

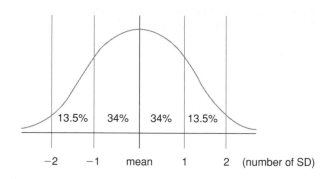

What is the mode? (2)
The most frequently occurring number.

In this type of distribution what can be stated about the values of the mean, mode, median and mid-range? (2)
They are identical.

Draw a distribution curve with a negative skew. (2)

Draw lines for the mean, mode, median and mid-range on it. (2)

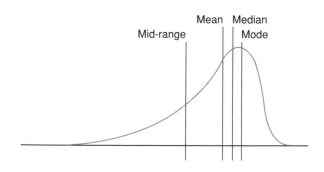

What is the formula for standard deviation? (2)

$$\sigma = \sqrt{\frac{\Sigma(x - \bar{x})^2}{N}}$$

where σ = standard deviation, Σ = sum of, x = the measured value, $\bar{x}$ = mean and N = degrees of freedom $(n - 1)$.

What is the formula for variance? (2)
Variance = the square of the standard deviation

What is the formula for standard error of the mean? (2)

$$SEM = \frac{\sigma}{\sqrt{N}}$$

where SEM = standard error of the mean, σ = the standard deviation and N = number of degrees of freedom $(n - 1)$

Easy, isn't it?

13. ANATOMY QUESTION

Oh no! Not pure anatomy again. I'll have to learn it!

This is an unmanned station. Look at this diagram and answer the following questions.

Name the dermatomes a-j indicated in the diagram. (10)

a. C2
b. C5
c. T1
d. C6
e. T1
f. T10
g. L1
h. L2
i. S1
j. S1

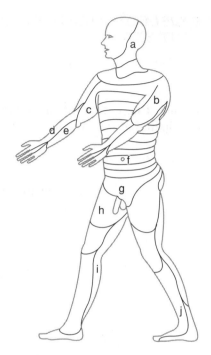

In checking the sensory level of spinal anaesthesia with a pin-prick, which dermatomal or segmental heights would you regard as adequate for the operations listed below?

Caesarean section(2)
T5.

Inguinal hernia repair (primary repair for an uncomplicated hernia)(2)
T10.

Haemorrhoidectomy(2)
S1.

Circumcision(2)
S1.

Open knee surgery(2)
L1.

14. DIAGNOSTIC/ELECTROCARDIOGRAM/ MANAGEMENT STATION

Occasionally some stations are combined to ask diagnostic and clinical information.

This station is unmanned. Please look at the following electro-cardiograph rhythm strip and answer the following questions.

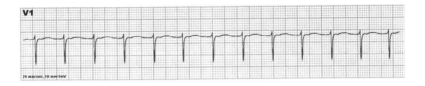

What is the rate of this strip? (2)
120/min.

Is it sinus rhythm? Why? (2)
No. There are no visible P waves.

The patient whose ECG is shown above, has no detectable carotid pulses. What is your diagnosis? (2)
Pulseless electrical activity (PEA).

What are the causes of this? (4)
The four Hs and four Ts as listed here: Hypovolaemia, Hypothermia, Hypo- or Hyperkalaemia, Hypoxia, Thrombo-embolism, Tension pneumothorax, Tamponade and Toxicity. *Yes! We know it's been in the previous paper but we wish to ensure that you know how important this is. Remember them!*

What drug of choice is indicated in the treatment of this condition? (2)
Epinephrine.

What dose would you give? (2)
1 mg.

How often would you give it? (2)
Every 3 min.

If the condition were associated with a bradycardia (<60/min) what drug and dose would you give? (2)
Atropine 3 mg intravenously.

What dose of this drug would you give down the tracheal tube? (2)
6 mg.

15. EQUIPMENT STATION

This is an unmanned station. This question is about pulse oximetry. Please answer the following questions.

What information does a pulse oximeter provide? (2)
It measures the oxygen saturation of the blood.

Describe how an oximeter works? (4)
Oximetry utilizes the different absorption coefficients of different wavelengths of light by oxyhaemoglobin and reduced-haemoglobin to measure oxygen saturation. At 660 nm wavelength (red light) reduced-haemoglobin exhibits an absorption approximately 10 times that of oxyhaemoglobin whilst at 940 nm wavelength oxyhaemoglobin exhibits the higher absorption.

Pulse oximetry operates with two alternating light emitting diodes and one sensing photo diode placed on opposite sides of a digit or any other suitable part of the body. It utilizes the isolation and processing of the pulsatile part of the signal of light absorption to verify the arterial component of oxygen saturation.

Draw an illustration showing the wavelengths used. (4)

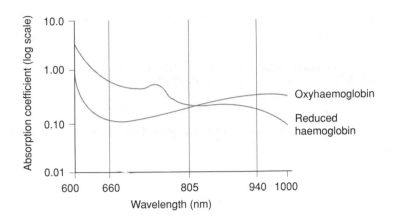

What is the 'isobestic point?'(2)
The isobestic point is the point at which two substances absorb a certain wavelength of light to the same extent. In oximetry it is 805 nm.

Give four examples of conditions where its measurement might be inaccurate. (4)
Four of the following. Causes of inaccuracies include: interference by ambient light, interference by diathermy, motion artifact, some types of dark nail varnish, measurements at low levels of saturation (below 80%), effect of different haemoglobin types such as methaemoglobinaemia, carboxyhaemoblobin, HbF and HbS, certain blood dyes such as methylene blue, and low perfusion states.

What could cause a trace like the one illustrated below? (2)

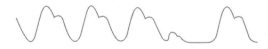

A premature extrasystole as evident from the timing of the wave signal and the reduction in its size.

When would you consider an oxygen saturation to be low? (2)
When it is less than 90%.

16. COMMUNICATION SKILLS STATION

Sometimes, as in real life, a relative gets agitated and even aggressive or tearful. The actors and actresses in the examination will behave the same way. You may find yourself insulted by a relative as in this scenario. An examiner will be present to observe and mark your performance.

Speak to the son of a 75-year-old man who is about to undergo surgery for the emergency repair of a ruptured aortic aneurysm. He is obviously anxious.
Introduce yourself and explain who you are and who the other members of the anaesthetic team are. Good afternoon. My name is Dr .... Please sit down. I will try to arrange some tea or coffee if you would like? I am one of the anaesthetists that will be looking after your father today (2). *No. I'll stand. You look very young! Are there some proper doctors around for me to talk too? I don't want to talk to you. Where's the consultant?* I am just one of the team looking after your father. The other doctors, including the surgeons are looking after your father now. They'll talk to you later. *They'd better!* I'm sorry to meet you in these circumstances but you need to know that surgery for a ruptured aortic aneurysm is major surgery. *What are you talking about? Speak my language!* Sorry. The aorta is the main artery that takes blood from the heart to the body and it is leaking (2). I'm sure you can see how important this artery is for the general health of us all. It can be repaired but the outcome depends upon how large the tear is, on where it is and what else is involved, and on the patient's general health (3). Before surgery can start we need to take some base line blood tests, and insert several monitoring device catheters so that he can receive the best possible care (2). The operation itself will take several hours whilst a graft is attached to the aorta. *Will my dad live?* We hope so. Often the outcome depends upon how easy this part of the surgery is. I'm sorry to say that occa-

sionally it can be impossible to do but normally it can be performed (3). *Incompetence more likely! Is the surgeon any good?* It is nothing to do with competence and the surgeon is a consultant. He is very skilled. I'll continue. Assuming surgery is successful your father will then be transferred to the Intensive Care Unit. He will be on a breathing machine until he is stable and he will need to be closely observed during this time. Of particular concern will be his kidneys and we shall need to monitor their function closely (3). Urine production is important, especially in this condition. You will be able to visit your father in the Intensive Care Unit but he will initially be sedated (2).

I shall keep you closely informed as to his progress but I need to inform you now that there is a significant mortality associated with this surgery. *You'd better save him. Mum needs him!* We'll be doing our best. However he has survived the initial bleed and therefore we are hopeful that he will do well (2). Any questions? (1)

Questions that may be asked by the relative may include the following: Will my father live? Can I see him now? Will he be in pain? Will he be aware? Should I get my brother here - he lives in America?

Thank you.

Be prepared for some pretty realistic acting in these clinical cases.

5 Sitting the examination and beyond

THE EXAMINATION

Preparation

To do well on the day of the examination itself, your brain needs to be primed and functional. Try and have a reasonable meal as your brain needs glucose and try and get a good night's sleep.

Some basic rules are worth repeating. Resist the temptation to relieve the tension the night before the examination by going out for a curry or drinking 12 pints of Newcastle Brown Ale. You may pay for it the next morning in the examination hall (so may the other candidates). If you're thinking of taking β-blockers, our advice is don't.

Sleep can be a major problem at this time. Often anxiety manifests itself as difficulty sleeping. Don't take pills! Accept it and try and sleep. Everyone is the same and sleeps badly, acquires gastro-enteritis on the day, and has their tongue stuck to their mouth at the start of the vivas and OSCEs.

As far as revision is concerned, some candidates have that 'bandanna-round-the-head', 'it's-not-all-over-till-it's-over' approach, and carry on ploughing through their revision plan through breakfast, on the train, even on their bicycle and stop only when they have to go into the examination itself. Others give up a day or two before ('If I don't know it by now . . .') and try to relax in advance. This is such a personal thing that there really is no ideal course; a compromise is to take the middle road and try to get one last night's good revision, but also try to flick through a few basics on the morning of the examination. It is actually quite easy to retain the odd extra fact for an hour or so and there's the added advantage of breaking the monotony of examination preparation whilst still giving your hands something to do. If you've slipped and haven't been going through your list of useful numbers and formulae as suggested previously, now might be a good time to try and learn two or three items.

On the day

Despite the fact that your nerves will be jangling somewhat, it is important that you try to get in a reasonable breakfast, since you'll be burning up energy rather faster than usual. If you're one of those people who express their anxiety by re-living their breakfast backwards, then at least drink something and take a few high-energy snacks with you. Make sure you leave home in good time; you don't want to arrive hot and sweaty, flustered, and certainly not late. Today is not the time to try an untested route into town or those new roller blades you were given as a birthday present. In general, it's probably best not to drive, since traffic and parking can be erratic, and there's nothing worse than driving around desperately looking for a parking space knowing that you're running out of time.

Nobody really cares what you look like for the MCQ examination, and there's a sort of unspoken competition amongst some candidates to see which one of them can look the most sleep-deprived, red-eyed and generally bedraggled. What you want is something comfortable; loose and light are generally good. Dress becomes particularly important for the oral examinations, of course, and despite all the best intentions for allowing individual expression and discouragement of stereotypes you simply must tow the line and wear suitable clothes. It is a professional examination. For men, this means suits; dark colours and traditional styles create the right impression. Beards and hair should be neat and tidy, clean-shaven faces should be clean-shaven. Women too have to dress the part; anonymity is the goal for you as well, although in a way it's harder since you are more likely to be accused of dressing up to create an advantage over your fellow candidates. Stereotypes run deep despite our attempts to view the world as fairly as possible. One last word about dress: oral examinations are notoriously hot and sweaty affairs so you're probably better off wearing something relatively cool and risking being cold than overheating and lighting up like a boiled beetroot.

Assuming you do arrive early, you'll have time to chat with fellow candidates, get a few more calories on board, and get into a positive frame of mind.

The MCQ examination

The MCQ examination is generally straight forward: you go in, sit down, arrange your equipment on the desk and wait for the instruction to start. Take off your watch and place it at the front of your desk, and make sure again that you know how much time you've got. The examiner will announce the rules and time limits, and tell you when to start, at which time you must turn over the question sheet and try to repress the wave of panic that usually follows. From then on, it's a matter of getting on with it. If you feel you simply cannot cope, stop for a minute (time yourself and count 60 seconds) and concentrate on your breathing, before going back in to join the fray. Whatever happens, keep an eye on the time and if you do run out of time, leave at least 15 minutes for transposing your answers to the optical reader card. Finally, make sure your number is correctly written on the answer sheet.

The time between the MCQ and oral examinations

After the MCQ try and clear your mind of matters relating to the examination, and put off your revision for a week or so.

Some candidates try to jot down every question they can remember for their colleagues and themselves to go over later, either to help others in the future or to see how they did (an agonizing process of rather dubious benefit). Others are either too exhausted to do this or don't see the point. The examiners naturally enough are not too keen on this practice, but everyone knows there is a large pool of apparently authentic questions floating around various anaesthetic departments.

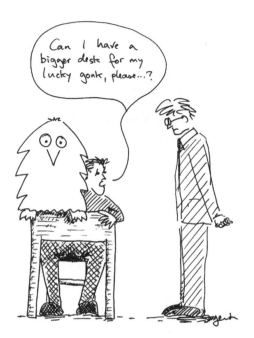

However you spend that week though, you must get back up to speed with your revision, only this time with a different slant to your initial written-orientated revision schedule. Viva practice is the crucial element now and you must nag every suitable member of your department to give you viva practice at every possible opportunity.

The oral examinations

In those last few moments before the examination starts, it's especially important to blow your nose, check your flies (and whatever the female equivalent is) and make sure there isn't a sprig of broccoli hanging from the corner of your mouth. Once things get going, the candidates tend to be herded around like sheep from viva to viva, which is probably a good thing since it removes one element of conscious thought and decision making. The reason for this regimentation is that the oral examination is extremely well organized and has to run smoothly for it to work, so you should just do as you're told and concentrate on your behaviour.

Remember, there are two examiners at each viva and one or two at each OSCE station. There may also be actors at OSCE stations, and the OSCE hall is usually full of assorted helpers and examiners wandering about making sure everything is running according to plan. You may also notice observers who have come to see how things are done and should take no part in the actual examination – don't try and involve them in the discussion at all as they will be trying to avoid interfering. If you come face to face with an examiner or observer who knows you, he or she should get up and swap places with someone at a different station, so that everything is correct and above board.

Immediately before the oral examinations start there is a huge fear factor – everyone feels ill, their hearts pound and the feeling of despair is enormous. Be reassured – it vanishes with the first question. By now you've hopefully improved your body language and people skills, but it's worth repeating a few things to yourself just before you meet the examiners for the first time. Be polite and courteous; say 'good morning/afternoon' at the start and 'Thank you' at the end. Remember that most impressions are made within the first five minutes of meeting you so make those 5 minutes your best performance. Resist the urge to run weeping from the room, no matter how badly you think you are doing. The examiners know how stressful the examinations are and will try to help you through, but you must let them help you. Look grateful at the appropriate moments and nod wisely when acknowledging their input.

In the time between vivas/OSCEs, make sure you check your appearance again but otherwise try to relax as much as possible. If any of your colleagues invite you to join them for a big lunch, ignore them.

One feature of the oral examinations is that after a whole day's traipsing around and being grilled, you then have to sit around waiting for the examination results, which are posted on a notice board at the end of the day.

WHAT NEXT?

If you pass

You'll feel great, no doubt about it. And why not, you've got over a significant hurdle in your career and an anaesthetic career beckons. A brief period of letting down your hair and enjoying life would seem entirely appropriate. The obvious next move is to plan your assault on achieving a specialist registrar post, and passing the Final Fellowship. It may be a time to catch up with home commitments, job movements and other features of life. Do consult with your College Tutor.

If you fail

Whoops! It happens to the best of us! It can be a crushing blow, whether expected or not, and you may experience the classic feelings of shock, anger and depression before finally coming to terms with it. You do need to find out which part(s) of the examination brought you down (details of your performance in the various parts of the examination will be sent to you by post) and talk about the way you handled them, and how well you thought they went at the time, with a trusted more senior colleague. It may be possible to identify specific areas of weakness and concentrate on them next time around. Any unsuccessful candidate may write to the Examinations Director of the Royal College for the actual marks attained in the written papers, and the comments and reasons for failure which were noted during the orals (individual examiners should never be contacted).

Two failures or a paper scoring marks of 1 in all parts results in an 'offer' of a mandatory guidance session at the Royal College, at which the candidate's actual papers will be gone through. This session is intended to be non-intimidating and The College is both serious about this and willing for the unfortunate candidate's trusted consultants and/or College Tutor to attend if requested. A confidential report from the candidate's College Tutor (with the candidate's permission) is also requested.

On a positive note, the additional period of revision required for further attempts at the primary examination will increase and consolidate your knowledge, which can only be an advantage when you come to start revising for the final fellowship . . . and look on the bright side – at least you have this book to help you prepare for the next attempt!

Index

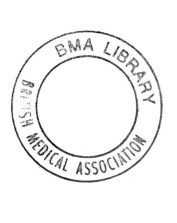